THE MEDICOLEGAL MIND

THE MEDICOLEGAL MIND

DAVID A F MORGAN

Copyright © 2024 by David A F Morgan.

Library of Congress Control Number:		2024915213
ISBN:	Hardcover	979-8-3694-9706-7
	Softcover	979-8-3694-9707-4
	eBook	979-8-3694-9705-0

All rights reserved. No part of this book may be reproduced or transmitted in any form or by any means, electronic or mechanical, including photocopying, recording, or by any information storage and retrieval system, without permission in writing from the copyright owner.

Any people depicted in stock imagery provided by Getty Images are models, and such images are being used for illustrative purposes only.
Certain stock imagery © Getty Images.

Print information available on the last page.

Rev. date: 08/28/2024

To order additional copies of this book, contact:
Xlibris
AU TFN: 1 800 844 927 (Toll Free inside Australia)
AU Local: (02) 8310 8187 (+61 2 8310 8187 from outside Australia)
www.Xlibris.com.au
Orders@Xlibris.com.au
859184

I dedicate this work to my Family.

FOREWORD

The legal and the medical professions each has its disparate skills, principles of practice, and theoretical lines. Complications arise when the two meet in a conflict, sometimes both as to fact and opinion.

This medicolegal arena calls for special attributes, suitable to its ends of determining the true facts relating to medical matters, both factual and theoretical, concerning a patient. The medical witnesses provide this evidence, as led and tested by the lawyers, according to relevance. The central role of the medical witnesses is plain.

To do it properly through a clear understanding of a duty to assist the Court by full, accurate and objective evidence is essential.

This work, reflecting a profound knowledge, understanding and experience of what is required of a medicolegal witness, brings out brightly the challenges and their proper responses required in a very practical, and even, it must be said, entertaining way.

I have thoroughly enjoyed reading its draft, and, without qualification, I support its advice.

The Honourable Desmond Derrington
B.A., LlB., LlD. (Honoris Casua), K.C..

PREFACE

This book distils my lessons, reflections, ruminations and experiences as an orthopaedic surgeon with an early and unrelenting interest in the medicolegal arena. Its stimuli are many and include my own motorcycle accident when I was 17 years old, and my subsequent education in medicine. I also have many friends in the Law. It was an easy fit.

Its origin is my newsletter, published monthly for about five years, with three sections; a lead article, a case vignette and some (humbly offered) general advice.

I have retained this format purposely. Its concept is that you will have the book beside your bed. You will read a chapter or two, before retiring. Not every night of course - just Mondays to Thursdays. Friday, Saturday and Sunday nights will be exempt. I hope that's when you'll be with family and friends enjoying good food with wine.

I genuinely hope that you enjoy it.

David A F Morgan
OAM, B.Sc.(Med)., MB., BS.(Hons)., F.R.A.C.S., F.R.C.Ed.(Orth)., F.A.Orth.A., C.I.M.E..

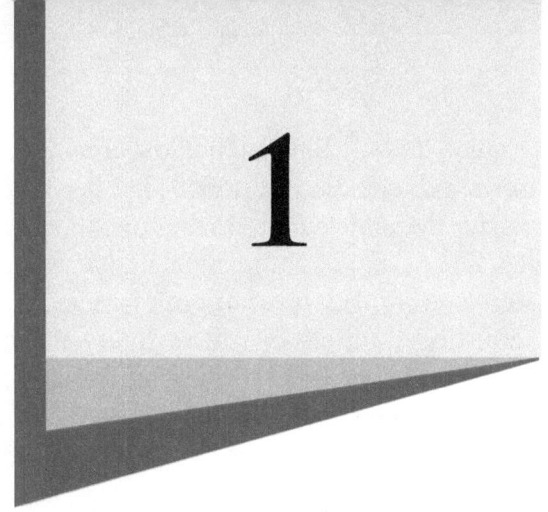

LEAD ARTICLE

Causation versus Liability in Personal Injury Litigation

It is best to be clear at the outset. A medical expert can assist in determining the presence or otherwise of causation of an injury, and perhaps the nature of that cause to a large or less degree. Conversely, liability for that injury is strictly a legal issue that is best left to the lawyers.

There are several important factors required to assess a causal link between an alleged injury and a compensable outcome. They comprise the gleaning of a thorough history, a complete physical examination, a review of ancillary investigations, and ultimately the making of a diagnosis that is based logically and demonstrably on those factors. It is then possible to retrace those steps and to provide an opinion on whether the alleged incident could have caused it.

Some exaggerated examples make it easy to understand.

A Motor Vehicle Accident

Imagine a patient, a driver who had been seated in a stationary car that was struck from behind by a following vehicle. The impact was minimal, as evidenced by the relevant slightly broken plastic taillight cover that had a minor crack and was replaced at a total cost of eighty-four Australian dollars. She had not lost consciousness, had not been trapped in the vehicle, did not notice that her seat was broken, and was able to drive the vehicle for a further one thousand kilometres on that same day. She never sought medical assistance for her alleged injuries. Her later claim for fractures of both femora, both tibiae, and both fibulae, requiring multiple operative interventions, prolonged hospitalization, and expensive and protracted rehabilitation plainly have no causal nexus with the accident that has been described. Whilst their cause may be uncertain, it can be stated with authority that they did not occur in the subject accident. The essential issue is cause.

Fall at a Building Site

At the other end of the spectrum, on the evidence of a claimant, supported by that of an independent witness, he fell from the seventh storey of a high-rise building, landing in an upright posture on a concrete pavement. He required life-saving resuscitation at the scene and was then transported to a major hospital for complex orthopaedic surgery to stabilize fractures in all bones of both lower limbs. Whilst stranger alternative causes have probably happened, it would be reasonable to attest to strongly probable causation between the fall and his injuries.

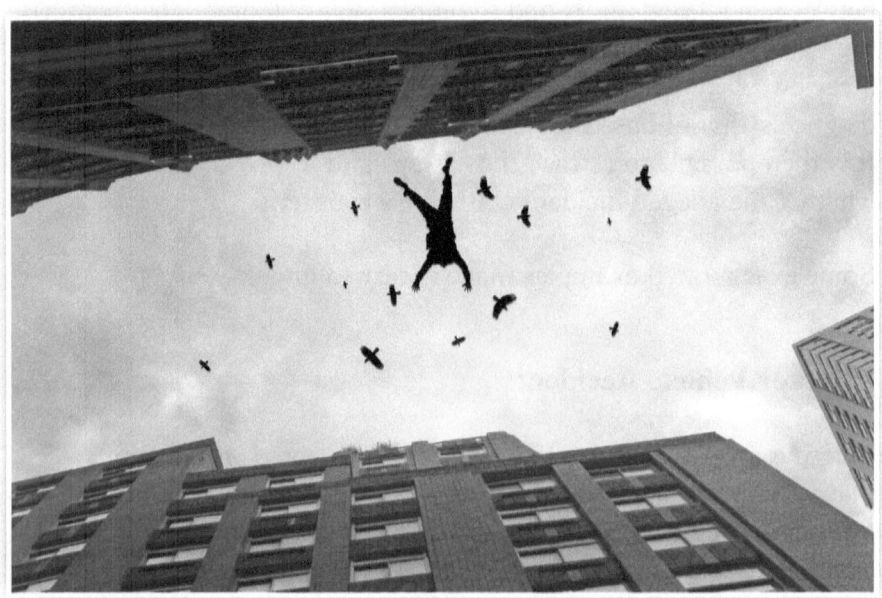

The Difficult Middle Ground

Unfortunately, most personal injury claims and allegations of medical negligence fall somewhere between these two obvious extremes, and then it is more difficult to assess causation. From a legal perspective, it is best if the medical expert can provide a definitive opinion whether a causal link exists, with a clear description of the competing factors and their strength, and the degree of their persuasion to the expert. The expert's balanced explanation for favouring one opinion over alternatives is most significant. Clarity of that explanation and confidence in the ultimate outcome are directly proportional. It is helpful for the court if an expert can nail her or his colours to the masthead by way of the expression of a conclusion with details that will assist the court in its determination on the whole of the evidence.

If it is not possible to be definitive, all differing options for interpretation, with suitable detail, should be provided to the court by way of assistance.

The expert's evidence should be balanced, complete, and clear.

CASE VIGNETTE

Whiplash, Whiplash, Whiplash …

I hate the term "whiplash"! It conjures up a vision of a rodeo performer in chaps, standing in the middle of a heavily hoof-marked, sandy ring and flailing a whip above his head. As he suddenly reverses direction on this beautifully woven leather device, a loud cracking noise splits the air. It really is quite dramatic. It is also an overstatement of what usually occurs at a clinical level in most rear-end collisions.

A better, albeit more complex and less sensational, expression would be a "flexion extension acceleration injury" or a "lateral flexion acceleration injury," which is really what commonly occurs in, respectively, a rear-end or T- boning motor vehicle collision.

Musculoligamentous strain injuries can ensue. It is also possible that there could be a derangement of one or more of the intervertebral discs, and a fracture could be sustained.

Consider This Lady

In this vignette, a sixty-three-year-old lady was a passenger in a Commodore sedan being driven by her husband. It had been stationary in a line of traffic at a set of traffic lights for more than thirty seconds when it was struck from the rear by a following four-wheel-drive vehicle fitted with a towbar and towing a trailer filled with concrete blocks. The forces were sufficient to shunt the Commodore sedan into the rear of the vehicle in front of it and damage it beyond economical repair. The lady lost consciousness briefly, and the squab of her seat was broken back to a horizontal level.

Under normal circumstances, it would be reasonable to expect that the patient sustained a very severe injury as a result of the contortion of her body through the impact to her vehicle, that it was of a compensable degree, and that any ongoing clinical attention was linked with the injury.

The Past History Is Important Too

A careful investigation of her history revealed that this was her fourth such accident of this nature and that she had already been compensated for the three previous ones.

Fortuitously, only weeks prior to this accident, she had undergone a careful, objective orthopaedic examination. That examiner had an opportunity to re-examine her twelve months following this accident, and he found little or no difference in her condition in the examinations.

It might be reasonable to conclude, therefore, that although her discomfort at the time of the accident may have been considerable, she had returned to her pre-accident state through natural progress.

Any ongoing measurable impairment should more likely be attributable to her three antecedent accidents rather than this last one.

If compounding harm is caused by successive independent events, one relevant to the proceedings and the rest not, apportionment of causal blame is very important.

GENERAL ADVICE

Which Documents Should Be Forwarded to the Medicolegal Reporter?

In essence, send everything. That may mean that there will be some extraneous material through which the reporter must wade, but it is better to have too much than too little. It sometimes happens that the relevance of some material to the reporter is not recognized by the sender, who is usually not an expert on the issue.

Radiographic examinations are especially important. Unfortunately, there is a move towards the supply of images on compact discs or online digital portals. There are several forms of software that will allow the images to be viewed. Almost every examination is accompanied by a preamble and warning. The warning states specifically, "These images are not intended for diagnostic purposes." You might well ask, "Well, what are they intended for?" That would be an excellent question.

It can be very frustrating to quality service to have a file that is either non-functional, incomplete, or corrupted.

Whenever possible, hard copy radiographs are preferable. It is not always possible, but every attempt to provide them should be made. They are becoming rare.

When issues of apportionment of blame or even negligence arise, it is useful also to have radiographs depicting the state of the anatomical segment that has been injured or disabled prior to the subject event. That enables the reporter to make a direct comparison between the respective states prior and subsequent to the event. This can also shed light on whether a duty of care to a vulnerable party was breached, and if so, it can be further assessed to see if that breach has resulted in an adverse outcome.

In summary, when preparing a file for forwarding and review, don't forget the radiographic component. It is of vital importance.

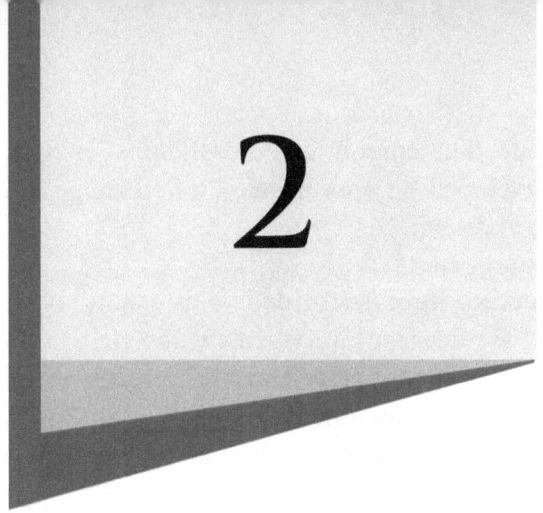

LEAD ARTICLE

Impairment Assessments—When, How, and Why?

Impairment relates to a loss, loss of use, or derangement of a body part, organ system, or organ function. It includes objectively identifiable impairments such as those due to a fracture, or those that are more subjective and may manifest themselves through fatigue or pain. Whilst both facets are important, it would be unwise to measure an impairment based on an analysis of the subjective feature alone.

Impairment Or Disability?

The term *impairment* is sometimes confused with *disability*. *Disability* has historically referred to the condition of a broad category of individuals with diverse limitations on their ability to meet social, occupational, domestic, or recreational demands. In essence, a disability is an alteration of an individual's capacity to meet personal requirements, whilst an impairment may be the feature that underpins it. The two are quite distinct.

The legal system dealing with compensation for personal injury caused by civil wrong allows the court to award special damages for identifiable and calculable losses, such as medical expenses and loss of wages, past and future, and general damages, which apply to such matters as pain and suffering, impairment and disability, and loss of enjoyment of life. The amount of general damages is at large, but the courts have developed an appropriate limited range in which general comparisons are drawn.

Many jurisdictions have a defined a threshold of say $250,000. The award is based on an injury scale value (ISV), which in turn is linked with an impairment assessment (a percentage of whole-person function) that can be quantified by an expert observer. The more precise the calculation, the more accurate the outcome.

Different jurisdictions use different guidelines for the calculation of this impairment. For example, it may relate to an individual body part. Ultimately, when multiple impairments are combined, a whole-person impairment (WPI) can be calculated, though not necessarily by simple addition where there may be overlapping. A patient without any impairment will exhibit a 0 per cent WPI. At the other end of the spectrum, the impairment might be a 99 per cent loss of whole-person function. This would be a quadriplegic who retains intellectual capacity and who, whilst incapable of any voluntary movement, would retain the insight of being trapped within one's own body. Most plaintiffs will fall somewhere between these two extremes.

Differing Guides For Evaluation

Several guidelines can be used. Those most referred to internationally are published by the American Medical Association in "Guides to the Evaluation of Permanent Impairment" (5th Edition) ("the AMA 5 Guides").

Previous iterations 1 to 4 have been historically well regarded. The sixth (6th) edition has been published, but adoption has been slow. It is not an improvement on the fifth (5th) edition and contains some inaccuracies.

Workers' compensation insurance authorities usually publish their own "Guides for the Table of Injuries". In that field, lawyers, medical experts, and Tribunals are expected to adhere to the norms laid down by these publications. Updates are introduced every few years.

The Department of Defence relies upon Comcare Tables, and other jurisdictions sometimes specify even more exotic tomes.

Whatever the required reference sourced it is incumbent upon the medical expert to use it wisely and accurately. Anything less should be avoided.

CASE VIGNETTE

The Unstable Back

Spondylolisthesis is a term which refers to the forward slippage of one vertebral body on the subjacent vertebral body. "Spondylo" is from ancient Greek and refers to the spine, and "listhesis" refers to the slippage or sliding.

There can be many causes. One is a defect or "fracture" that occurs in the lower part of the lumbar spine. Approximately 1% of the population can be born with it in the pars interarticularis. A further 3% or 4% will develop it over the following three or four years of life. It follows that 4% or 5% of the normal population six years or older will have this defect.

A subset of this population will then develop the forward slippage of one of the affected vertebrae on the subjacent vertebra. This is called a "lytic spondylolisthesis".

Despite the dramatic appearance of these changes on radiographs of the vertebral column, most of these patients remain asymptomatic and are not aware of the presence of the condition.

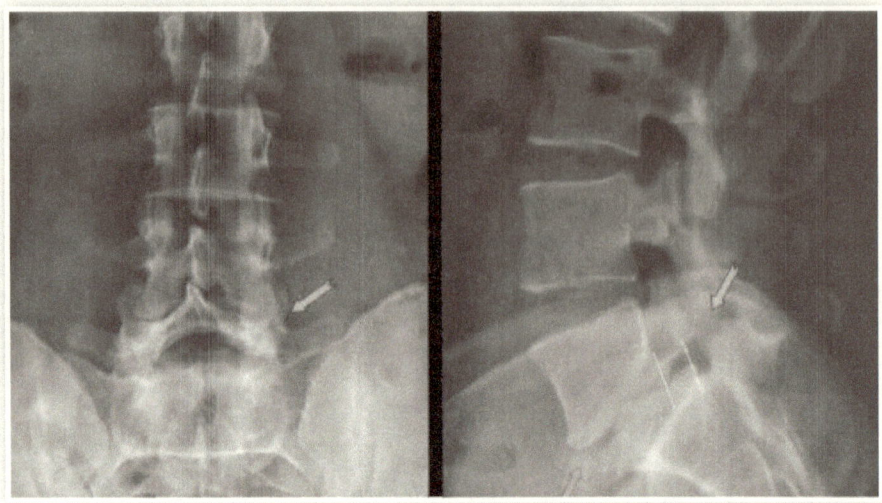

The top arrows depict the pars interarticularis defect. The bottom arrow indicates the forward slippage of L5 on S1

They can also be subjected to injuries in the workplace. Radiographic examinations reveal the underlying problem and stimulate great interest from all concerned. There is a temptation to attribute this ongoing clinical symptom complex to this underlying condition and ignore the effects of a workplace accident.

A further small subset will be aware of back problems. They suffer from degeneration of the disc between the two mobile vertebral segments. These changes are often apparent on plane radiographs with narrowing of the disc space and other degenerative changes. They cause back ache after activity and stiffness after rest.

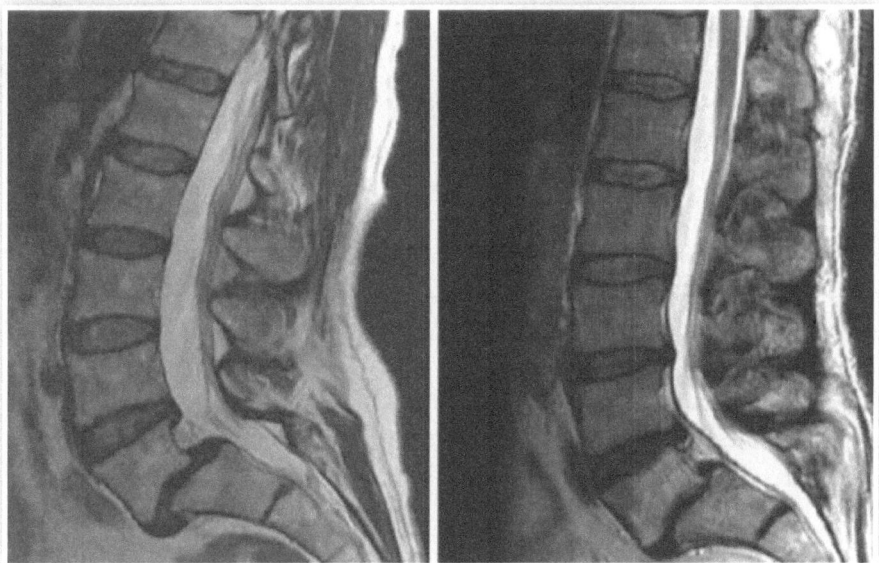

This CT scan shows how the cauda equina and nerve roots can be compromised

Is The Spondylolisthesis Relevant?

Careful analysis is required. If the patient was truly asymptomatic prior to the accident and there are no indications to the contrary, it might be reasonable to conclude that the accident under investigation caused any ongoing clinical circumstance. But if it can be demonstrated with confidence that the antecedent condition had been symptomatic prior to the accident, the accident may have given rise to either nothing more than a temporary exacerbation or alternatively, a permanent aggravation of the pre-existent condition. Apart from the issue as to the anticipated duration of the harm, apportionment of blame for any alteration will be necessary.

GENERAL ADVICE

Can The Expert's Mind Be Changed?

Yes. Special circumstances may apply.

Imagine a scenario where an expert's report does not align closely with the complaints made by the plaintiff, or with Counsel's own perception of the plaintiff's case in respect of 'facts' communicated to the expert.

The mismatch may result from the inadequate supply of relevant information, an unreasonable bias on the part of the expert or a true misunderstanding between perception and reality.

Not All "Facts" Are Facts

Every month or so, I am involved in a teleconference or a face-to-face meeting when lawyers acting for the opposing party test me upon my expressed views. This is a proper and appropriate exercise which I genuinely welcome. I enjoy the interchange. For various possible reasons, I am capable of error, and some complex processes require explanation. I am in pursuit of the correct conclusion.

I have not kept any statistics as to the likelihood of my changing my opinion. Its frequency is probably irrelevant. More importantly, the process should be applauded. A medicolegal analysis does not end with the furnishing of a report at the end of a consultation. It is a continuum which is likely to pass through mediation and possibly to trial and appeal. When accepting a brief, it is necessary to recognize its full potential extent, and that although the opinion given should be honest, clear and unambiguous, it could still be wrong. There may be occasions when I will have to "change my mind".

When?

There is a classic situation in the courtroom. Under cross-examination, a dogged expert with a rigid view, is presented with a new and established version of events and new facts. They contradict those forming the basis of his opinion. Asked to assume that they are true, nonetheless, "Dr Bombastic" resolutely refuses to budge. There is an adage that "nothing evaporates as quickly as yesterday's success". So be it with credibility.

There are times when the expert simply must and should acknowledge a previously expressed opinion to be incorrect. It can be done with grace and dignity, but not without proper and full consideration. The Court is not unaware of difficulties, and on appeal, judges themselves have been found to have been in error.

LEAD ARTICLE

Economic Losses Associated With Personal Injury and Medical Negligence

This is likely to be a big-ticket item in any claim based on injury suffered prior to retirement. It includes losses that have accrued to the time of judgment following an injury, and those that are likely to accrue in the future. The latter often has a larger element of speculation depending on medical factors. Their analysis may be complex and requires very special care and attention.

Many variables must be considered. The list includes the injured party's age and sex, level of education, prior work experience with or without trade qualifications, determination to improve, doggedness and stoicism together with the prevailing economic climate. Of course, any mention of this minimizing factor should be accompanied by a reference to the price that it would demand, for example in the form of suffering further pain.

A claim based on "total and permanent disablement" will require the expert to review the definition with particular care.

Economic loss and disability are very closely linked. Usually, economic loss and impairment may bear some, but less relationship.

For example, if an operating orthopaedic surgeon was to amputate the dominant upper limb through the mid- forearm level by a chainsaw, any ability to return to such work would be expected to be permanently lost. Single-handed surgery does not work! Conversely, if a barrister sustained a similar injury, she or he could return to work in due course, albeit with the bandaged forearm in a sling, and with the aid of a clerk to write any notes.

Their impairments would be identical, but their disabilities would be dramatically different.

Another Example

A more realistic example may be found in the case of a 40-year-old tree lopper who has sustained a severe injury involving one or more lumbar intervertebral discs requiring operative intervention, including decompression and stabilization of the vertebral column. He has been away from work practices for 18 months. He attended high school to year 9 level only, and has no trade qualifications or work experience other than that associated with the construction industry. In particular, he has no clerical, office or administrative skills.

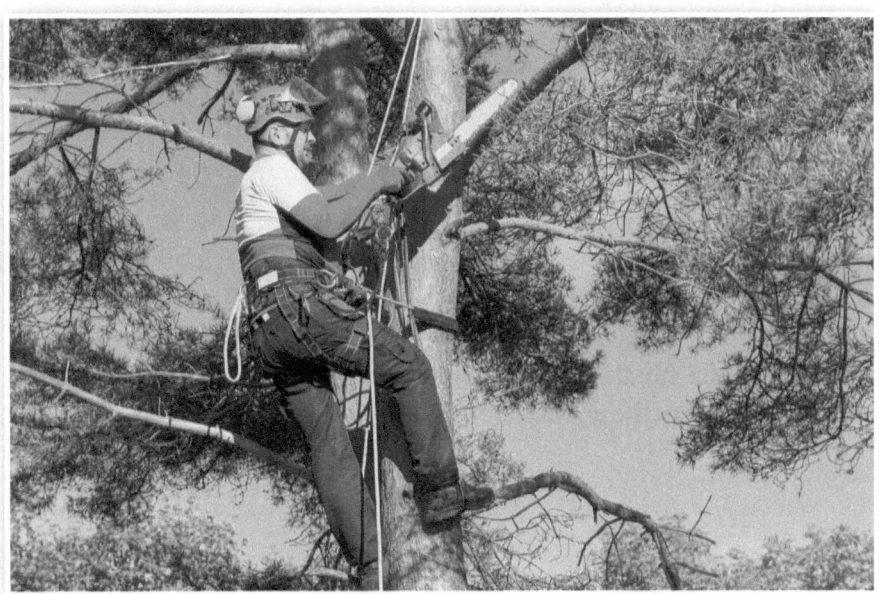

Because of the severity of his disability, it would be unrealistic to expect him to return to work as a hands-on arborist. Considerable losses of wages could be expected in the future, in addition to those already incurred through his inability to return to work.

It may be possible, however, that a suitable retraining programme may equip him with some skills that would allow him to secure remunerative work until he has reached a reasonable retirement age. It may, for example, allow him to work as a telemarketer, as a call centre operator or even as a factory worker in a seated position performing light bench work. It would be necessary to consider that he would need to sit or stand at will during a working day but nonetheless, he could be productive.

Making The Correct Decision

Given the importance of this facet of any personal injury or medical negligence claim, it is imperative that the assessing expert addresses all variables in a transparent and cogent manner. A clear and concise explanation of an opinion may assist the Court to quantify the losses with much greater accuracy.

CASE VIGNETTE

Just How Innocuous Is A Tibial Fracture?

A 17-year-old boy wearing shorts and boots on a work experience programme at a cattle station in the Northern Territory fell from a horse. He sustained a fracture of his left tibia (shin bone). Clinical examination found a 1cm laceration over the mid third of the shin, at the level of the tibial fracture. He was air lifted to a major hospital, underwent an orthopaedic operation and the wound was closed primarily.

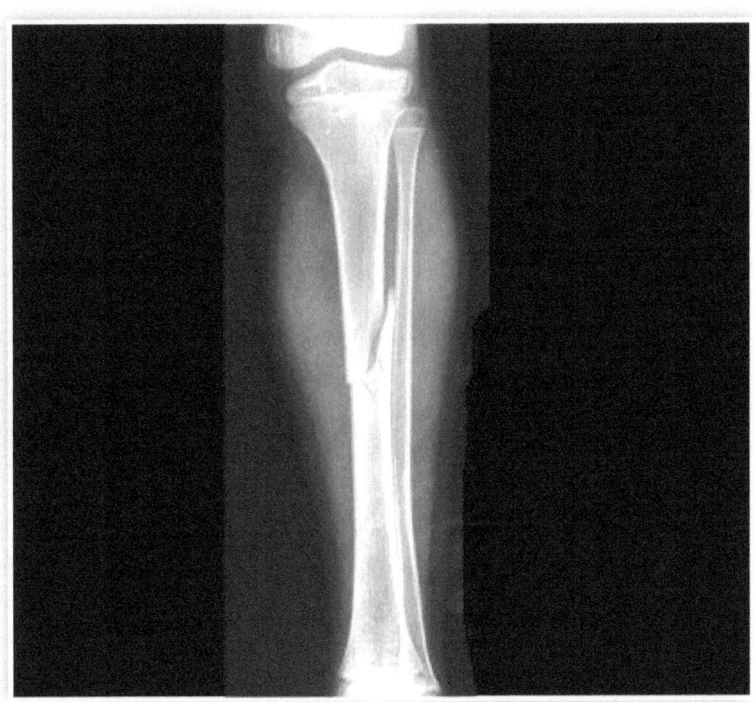

An isolated tibial fracture

The accident occurred on a Tuesday. By Saturday, he had to have a below-knee amputation.

So What Happened?

In the intervening four days, he developed gas gangrene; an overwhelming infection caused by the bacterium Clostridium *welchii* or *perfringens*. It is a bacterium that is found in many locations, including livestock faeces. As he had suffered a compound fracture, it is probable that a spike of bone had pierced the skin and retracted spontaneously. The spike was presumably contaminated with enough material containing the Clostridium bacterium to produce an infection. This bacterium proliferates best in the absence of oxygen. Because the wound was closed, the tissue was devitalised (de-oxygenated) and any form of antibiotic therapy could not perfuse the region successfully, an ideal incubator for the bacterium was created. Over the next forty-eight to seventy-two hours, an overwhelming and life-threatening infection developed. It was either remove the limb or lose his life.

When he was being examined for medicolegal purposes, I recall his being incredulous. He'd been offered a position in an Australian Rules Football gifted player programme. In the space of a week, that career had evaporated.

This was a particularly salutary experience for all involved. Had the wound been left open, adequate wound toilet been performed, and the incubation environment not been created, a much more satisfactory outcome may have been achieved.

So, we have personal injury both because of the work environment AND possible medical negligence. This will be an interesting case.

GENERAL ADVICE

The Expert In Court – How To behave?

Respectfully! And hoping for professional respect, but with calm dignity and rational response if it is not forthcoming. Remember that Counsel's aggression, when it is present, is not personal, but mostly in answer to the demands of the efficient performance of the task. If it is gratuitous, the Court is usually aware of that Counsel's predilections, and makes adjustments. Some Counsel can be quite barbarous in cross examination, but that, if gratuitous, is usually recognized as compensating for a lack of talent.

Just as legal professionals are likely to feel uncomfortable in an operating theatre (whether as a patient or as an observer), so do most medical experts feel uncomfortable in a Court room. It is a concept alien to them to relinquish control and be under scrutiny and direction.

The Expert's Armour and Shield

It is best that the expert has initially produced an objective, transparent and easily understandable medicolegal opinion. It should be full in the form of describing facts and features that might support a competing view, accompanied by reasons as to why one should be preferred. It is also desirable to remain patient and calm and not respond to barbs with equal aggression. The expert should not be polarised but should view the role as assisting the Court in its understanding of matters within his domain. The Court affords professional expert witnesses some considerable benefits and expects neutrality in return. It is not for them to influence, coerce, pre-empt or otherwise entertain.

Confidence with humility, clarity of thought, economical explanations and equanimity are all qualities of a competent expert witness.

I relish the opportunity to appear personally in Court because of its intellectual rigour. Telephone evidence is less disruptive but not so fulfilling. Mind you, I have experienced some very bumpy rides! It is commonly accepted that good Court room performance comes from experience. Unfortunately, some experience comes from poor Court room performance.

On one occasion, a cross-examiner repeatedly prefaced questions with "I put it to you …", which is a form of posing a proposition seeking agreement. The propositions were unsound. Rather than expressly disagreeing and explaining why they were wrong, I kept replying "Why" .. as if to say .. "Why would you put that to me?" The District Court Judge (a crusty old fellow, now deceased), interjected and told me to "Just answer the question!". In my naivety, I did not appreciate that I was being questioned. When the judgement was delivered, a barrister-mate sent me a copy. In referring to my evidence, the judge wrote … "he reminded me of a straggly, white -haired old professor who claimed 'there was a cup and a half of full cream milk in every bar of Cadbury's chocolate' ". Clearly, my evidence was not preferred! A valuable lesson!!

Another episode stands out too. I was being cross examined by a barrister who behaved much like a chameleon. Mostly she was pleasant and charming, but without warning she would flash her gums and be extremely aggressive. In retrospect, I became unsettled, and combative. In the ensuing judgement, my evidence was referred to as being "polarised and argumentative". Even though the side that had called me won the case, my evidence was dismissed.

Both "come-uppances" occurred over 2 decades ago. They have remained clear in my mind, and I strove to avoid repetition.

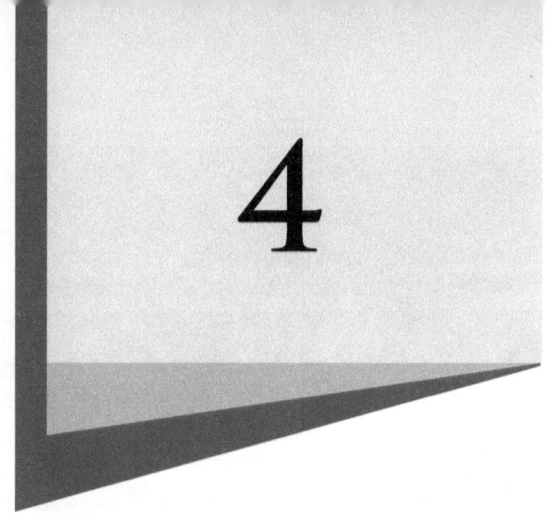

LEAD ARTICLE

Social And Recreational Activities

Whilst most attention in reports in personal injury and medical negligence claims focuses upon impairment or disability assessments, causation, economic loss, and future therapeutic needs, it is also usually necessary to assess losses of social and recreational enjoyment that are caused by a traumatic incident.

Some plaintiffs will have been extremely active before and until their respective injuries. A serious injury with ongoing impairments and disabilities may have permanently diminished or even destroyed their ability to return to some semblance of their former lifestyle.

A medical expert must be well positioned to assist with this analysis. Though the consequences of some injuries are totally irreversible, the adverse effects of others can sometimes be reduced quite significantly by the provision of splints, braces, orthoses and prostheses. A stiff, painful ankle could be splinted, allowing a return to some limited bush walking and hiking. Advice on modified techniques to accomplish tasks which were previously taken for granted may also be usefully provided. For example, the use of a motorised golf buggy may allow a previously keen golfer to make at least a limited return to that favoured pursuit.

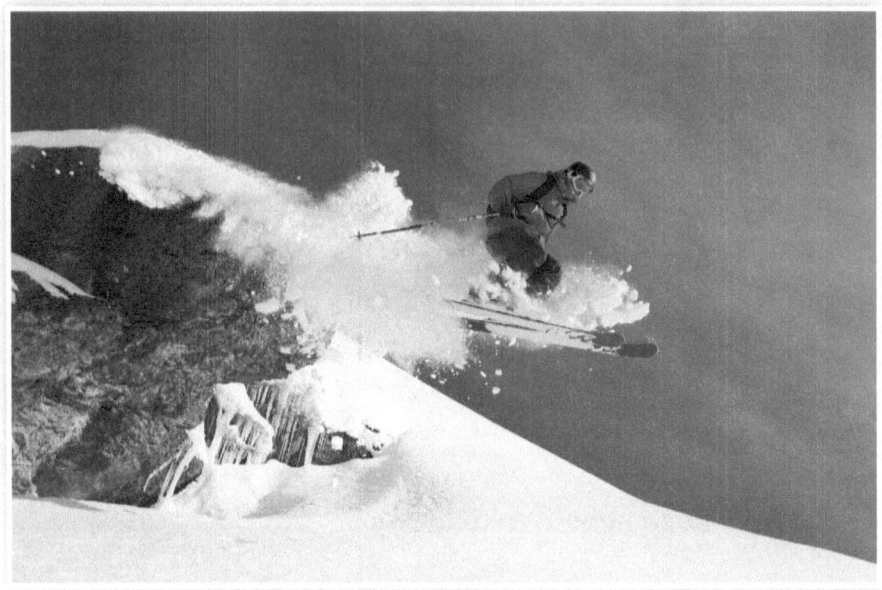

Addressing this important issue of social and recreational capacity is a serious part of any medico-legal report, which should not only describe the consequences that are present, but also refer to any available forms of amelioration that are or may be available, particularly if they are not yet being used.

Establishing an easy rapport facilitates the gleaning of these personal details. Some patients are more adaptable than others. Relatively trivial injuries may, to some, provoke major lifestyle changes.

It is important that the expert listens to the plaintiff, though not always accepting that information. Separating genuine complaints from self-serving exaggeration is equally imperative. We will all benefit from an expert who is experienced, sympathetic and realistic.

CASE VIGNETTE

But He Didn't Hurt His Ankle!

The plaintiff sustained a fracture involving the upper end of his shin bone. It was managed successfully; it had united without difficulty, and he was expected to return to an asymptomatic state.

His claim centred upon his ipsilateral (same side) ankle. He complained of pain, swelling and stiffness which would, he said, interfere with his ambulatory capacity and compromise his future economic prospects as a labourer.

Really??!

The insurer was incredulous. How was it that this upper shin fracture had given rise to such a debilitating problem with his ankle?

The therapeutic regimen had been of a non-operative nature, and merely involved the application of a long leg cast for four months. The cast had not been well applied, and the ankle was fixed in a downward position (plantar flexion) for that entire period. Secondary capsular contractures formed, and inadequate attention was paid to the problem following removal of the cast by the physiotherapist. At the end of an 18-month period, the ankle joint remained quite stiff, and the capsular contractures appeared to be solid.

Whilst uncommon, this is a recognised sequel to an inappropriate positioning of the joint for a prolonged period without proper rehabilitation. Although the ankle itself may not have been injured originally, the following sequence of events may render the ankle malady a part of the total harm caused by the original wrong and of compensable nature. The causative link is indirect but real. The medical misfeasance may be a concurrent cause involving claims for contribution between the tortfeasors. This is true unless it was found that the later medical negligence was independent of the original harm in a way that would confine the plaintiff's award to actions against the respective wrongdoers.

GENERAL ADVICE

Hysterical Orthopaedics

The word "hysteria" has specific psychiatric connotations. Patients who are thought to suffer with hysteria sometimes present with conversion disorders.

In the orthopaedic paradigm, patients may present with fixed contractures, for example of a hand or fingers, because of complete non-use for a protracted period. That period can be measured in years. As a result of holding the hand in a curled-up position across the front of the torso, permanent contractures can form, and the digits can simply not be extended. I have seen such a case.

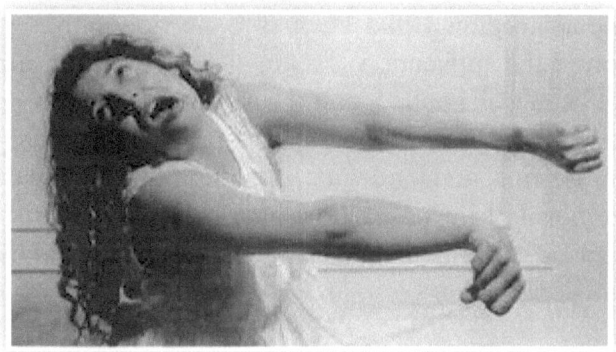

Fixed contractures of wrists and hands

How does it arise?

Although there may have been a precipitating injury, it may have been relatively minor. It may not have been in the class of injury that would result in such a devastating outcome. Rather than being of a physical origin, it is more likely to be of a psychiatric origin.

That does not mean that the patient is not impaired, nor does it mean that the patient is not seriously disabled. It simply means that the causative inciting agent has complex overtones other than those of a purely physical nature.

These claimants require a specialist psychiatric assessment.

LEAD ARTICLE

Future Therapeutic Costs – Who Pays What And When?

Plaintiffs undergoing a medicolegal examination have usually reached a state of Maximal Medical Improvement (MMI) following the index injury or incident. Many months and sometimes years have elapsed and the clinical recovery, regardless of its complexity, has usually plateaued.

Expenditures to date can be quantified precisely. That's the easy part. It is more difficult to assess future therapeutic requirements accurately. An insightful understanding of the natural history of conditions, an ability to predict a correct prognosis, and experience with all facets of medical costs are required.

Consider This

A 58-year-old lady has fallen at the shopping centre, but there is more to it than just a fall. She has sustained a fracture involving her proximal thigh bone or femur in the form of a femoral neck fracture (or NOF). Varying therapeutic regimens are available for managing this problem but one consists of a total hip replacement.

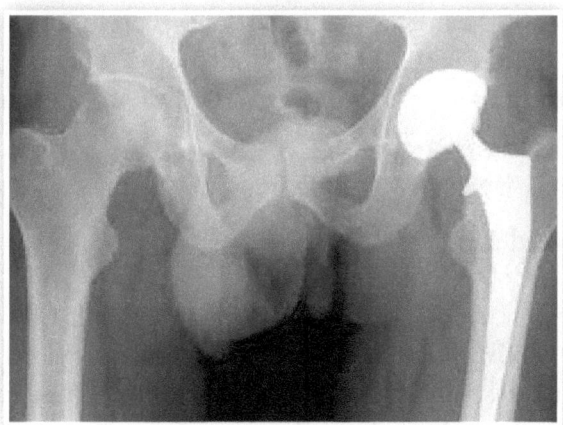
Left total hip replacement

Hip replacements perform superbly under normal circumstances. Those performed for femoral neck fractures are less successful but are still more than satisfactory.

The implanted medical devices are man-made and so, can wear, loosen, fracture and fail. It is a reasonable assumption that a hip replacement will not last "forever".

So How Long Will It Last?

This is difficult to predict in respect of a specific patient. Longitudinal studies of large population groups can give some statistical indication. If it's well performed, it has, on average, a 90% chance of not requiring revision within 20 years. It would be unrealistic to think that all will fail in their 21st year. Clearly, that is not the case. Many will last 30 years, some 40 years and there may even be a few still around in 50 years if the plaintiff lives long enough. We are all living longer.

If we come back to our 58-year-old plaintiff and given that she has a further life expectancy of about three decades, we can expect, statistically, that she has at least a 15% chance of requiring a revision operation at some future time. Revision hip replacements are more complex and more expensive than a primary hip replacement. Costs can be assessed variously but generally, a total expenditure in the vicinity of $60,000 can be expected. It may therefore be reasonable to allocate 15% of that $60,000 in her final award. That is for the Court, but it needs the benefit of reliable expert advice to inform it of what it does not know on these matters.

Costs Can Add Up

Other and less obvious costs can also be incurred. She may require the use of a walking stick or a wheelchair. She may need intermittent analgesics with associated pharmaceutical costs. These can become a very important part of any award or settlement of a personal injury or medical negligence claim. She may require physiotherapy and repeated visits with her local medical officer or her orthopaedic surgeon. All these factors require appreciation and informed speculative calculation.

CASE VIGNETTE

Is It The Shoulder Joint Or The Acromioclavicular Joint?

The shoulder joint is formed by the upper end of the arm bone (the humerus) and a socket (the glenoid) on the outer edge of the shoulder blade (the scapula). It is the humeral head which articulates with the glenoid process.

The acromioclavicular joint is nearby, but separate. It is formed by the outer end of the collar bone (the clavicle) and the inner aspect of the acromion (part of the shoulder blade but well above the socket). The shoulder girdle itself works synchronously but these two joints do remain separate. The acromioclavicular joint not uncommonly develops degenerative changes as patients age. The shoulder joint less so.

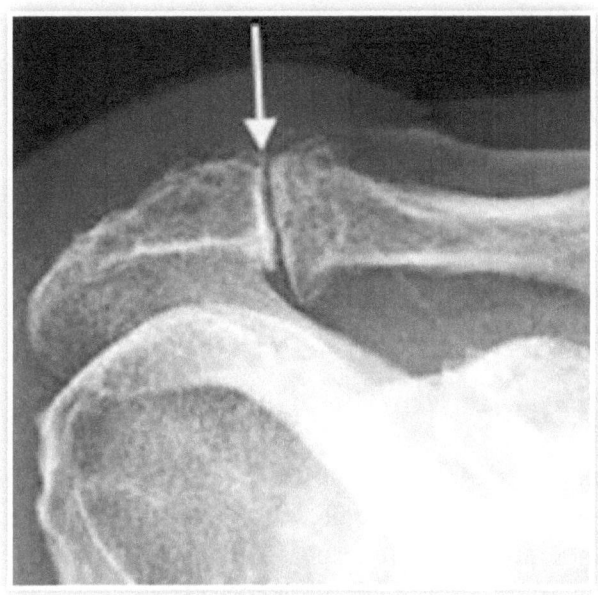

The arrow indicates the A-C joint

So What Is The Issue Here?

A plaintiff may be injured and sustain ongoing problems referable to the shoulder joint (glenohumeral joint) itself. This may involve the rotator cuff, the labrum around the glenoid, the glenoid itself or even the humeral head. Specific therapeutic regimens may be required, functional losses may result, and compensation could be due.

It should be appreciated however that the acromioclavicular joint is not necessarily involved in the process, and injury to it is often separate to the shoulder joint proper. During an operative management programme for the glenohumeral or shoulder joint, some upper limb surgeons will also ablate the acromioclavicular joint by removing the outer end of the clavicle.

That supplemental procedure is not necessarily linked with the original injury and is therefore not compensable. The AMA 5 Guides however ascribe some considerable importance to the acromioclavicular joint. The excision of the outer end of the clavicle, thereby ablating the acromioclavicular joint, yields a loss of 10% of upper extremity function or a loss of 6% of whole person function. Refer to Table 16-27 on page 506 and Table 16- 3 on page 439 to check these calculations. This is a significant impairment, but it is not necessarily due to the subject accident. Apportionment of blame will be necessary.

Insurers beware!

GENERAL ADVICE

Mandatory Reporting In The Medicolegal Setting

The national law governing health practitioners in Australia contains a subsection dealing specifically with mandatory reporting. Most western democracies have the same. This is where practitioners who are aware of some significant underperformance on the part of a colleague are obliged to report that underperformance for investigation and appropriate management. This most commonly occurs in a clinical setting such as a hospital or an environment where clinicians can observe each other. Occasionally, this can also arise in the medicolegal setting.

Consider This Scenario

I recall a telephone call from a colleague. He had seen a young woman who had sustained a seemingly relatively innocuous injury to a knee joint and who had been managed variously by three orthopaedic surgeons over a four-year period. The woman was in her late twenties and had undergone no fewer than twelve operations. It appeared that some of the operations were particularly unwise and possibly poorly performed. For example, the ninth operation was the performance of a total knee replacement. This would be a very uncommon operation for a woman in her late twenties who was otherwise relatively fit and well. The tenth and eleventh operations were aimed at eradicating overwhelming sepsis within the joint. The operations were poorly timed, ineptly performed and destined to fail. Unfortunately, the final operation was an above knee amputation.

The question posed by my colleague was how he should address the matter outside the medicolegal arena. It does pose a conundrum. Most of what he has become aware of was subject to legal privilege residing in the patient on whom he was providing a medical report. Perhaps he should remain quiet outside his medicolegal report? Conversely, by doing so, was he theoretically putting future patients at risk? I suggested he discuss the matter with the referring solicitor. Ideally, he would be released to notify the medical registration agency about his concerns. That is the body charged with investigations and sanctions. I'm not sure what he did.

Whilst my advice was circumspect and not definitive, I believed he had no option but to advise the regulator (in this case AHPRA or the Australian Health Practitioner Regulation Agency) of the sequence of events and leave it with them. Although I do not have total confidence in the system, there is no better avenue available. At least he could hope for a thorough investigation and appropriate action. Simply letting the matter rest is not my preferred option.

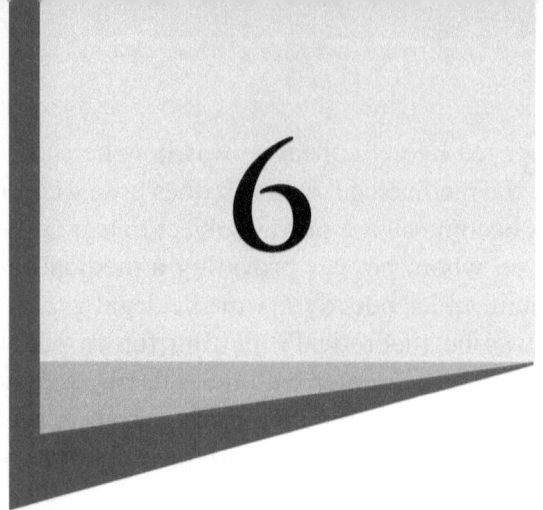

LEAD ARTICLE

Future Care Costs Can Be Significant

The sure can! They may become enormous.

Consider this example. A formerly, fit, well and active 20-year-old female has been rendered quadriplegic in a jet ski accident on a tropical island holiday.

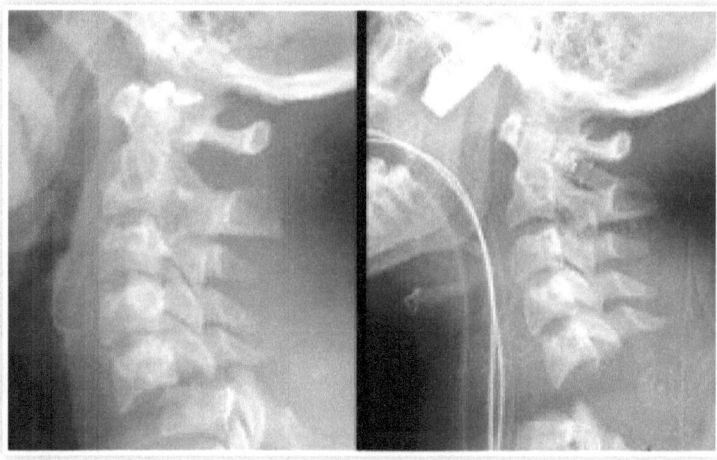

Complete spinal cord transection at C5-6

Despite all best intentions and the supply of the very latest of devices, she will be heavily dependent upon total and full-time care by family, friends, professionals and others for the remainder of her life. Enormous care costs are likely to accrue.

At the other end of the spectrum is a 50-year-old male who has sustained a fracture of his non-dominant wrist. It did not require any operative intervention and was managed satisfactorily with a plaster cast for eight weeks. Physiotherapy then led to gradual improvement, and he was eventually capable of most sedentary activities of daily living. He is a non-complaining plaintiff and from an outward perspective, appears to get on with his life without much difficulty.

Not All Is As It May Seem

Closer scrutiny reveals that he has significant restrictions in wrist movement, quite marked pain when his wrist is forced backwards or forwards and difficulties gripping objects. He cannot rotate his forearm sufficiently to grip an object with any authority.

Favoured activities such as lawn mowing, heavy gardening, trimming branches from overhead trees and cleaning leaves from the gutters around his house are now much more difficult. Whereas he would previously have accomplished these tasks without a second thought, he has now become dependent upon others for support. He is a bachelor, has no siblings, no relatives living nearby and is almost friendless. He will need to engage outside contractors to assist with all those seemingly menial tasks. Considerable ongoing costs are likely to accrue. The important "6 hours + a week" threshold might be exceeded. In the state in which I practice, if domestic assistance needs exceed this level, compensation is payable.

When assessing the costs of future domestic care, it is important for the expert reporter to assess the plaintiff's injury at an individual level. We all differ in our capacities, incapacities, and disabilities and in the availability of inexpensive aid. Precision in a report on this issue can come only from a thorough relevant investigation which can support a precise analysis.

CASE VIGNETTE

Knee Ligament Injuries

The knee joint is a most complex structure. It is capable of hinging, gliding and rotation. Attempts to reproduce this complex biomechanical event artificially have been met with less than total success. Nature's competence employs a special arrangement of ligaments both within and without the joint. The inside ligaments include the anterior and posterior cruciates. The former (anterior cruciate ligament or ACL) is not uncommonly torn in rigorous sporting activities such as football, netball and snow skiing because of the intense stress placed on the joint.

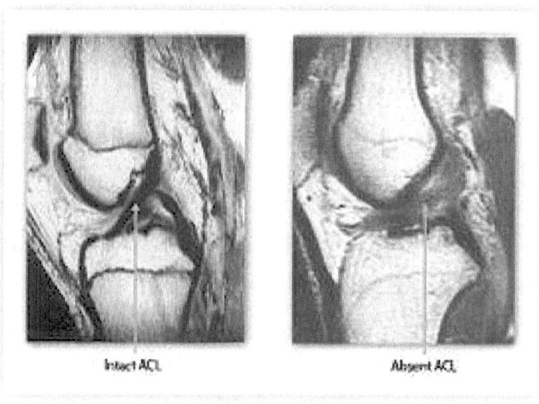

MRI scans of intact and torn ACL's

So What?

The cruciate ligament itself has a rich blood supply. When it is ruptured, the joint rapidly fills with blood. It is also associated with considerable pain. Over subsequent weeks, this haemarthrosis resolves and the injured knee gradually improves. Unfortunately, some patients suffer ongoing rotary instability. They can walk and even run in a straight line but their attempts to pivot or suddenly change direction are met with pain and a sensation of instability. The knee joint sometimes gives way.

Many of these require an operative reconstruction. The hamstring tendons can be harvested from the thigh, or the patellar tendon can be harvested from the front of the knee itself. Artificial ligaments are sometimes used, though with limited success. Allograft tendons (from deceased donors) also play a major role, especially in revision reconstructions.

A patient who has an ongoing cruciate ligament instability that has not been repaired, and who remains seriously symptomatic, will have suffered a loss of up to 10% of whole person function. This loss can be quantified using Table 17-33 on page 546 of the AMA 5 Guides. Even after a successful reconstruction, some patients will continue to exhibit mild ongoing instability amounting to a loss of 3% of whole person function.

This should attract a component of General Damages for pain and suffering. in addition, because of the ongoing instability, remunerative, recreational and domestic activities could be compromised. Further financial losses may accrue.

But Wait, There's More

The chronic instability may be a precursor to osteoarthritis. Over decades, the disease may progress so that a joint replacement is eventually required. Very considerable, unexpected costs can result.

What began as a seemingly innocuous knee injury, metamorphoses into an issue with lifelong ramifications. If this is a claimable event, it behoves the reporter to raise these possibilities to ensure full justice is done to the claimant.

GENERAL ADVICE

Differentiating Between Complications And Negligence

Negligence is a term used by lawyers and in that sense, it is not necessarily in the purview of medical practitioners. From the latter's perspective, the term relates to three interlinked activities. The first relates to a duty of care to the patient in the provision of treatment. It would be hard to deny that such a duty existed in a clinical liaison.

The second relates to a breach of that duty. From a medical perspective, this can be more difficult to analyse although expert opinions can assist.

The third is the establishment of a link between any breach and an adverse quantifiable outcome. Unfortunately, complications occur and could seemingly fall under the heading or guise of "negligence". "Doctor, you amputated the wrong leg!".

Let us look at some adverse outcomes. More than 50,000 Australian patients undergo total hip replacement every year. This is an extraordinary number of operative interventions and almost all of them do extremely well. A small but finite percentage does not do well. Almost 1% of patients will have an infection. Of those, 2% or 3% will note ongoing sepsis indefinitely. A further 1% or so may suffer a dislocation of the joint. Again, a small subset of that 1% may have recurrent dislocations and require further operative intervention.

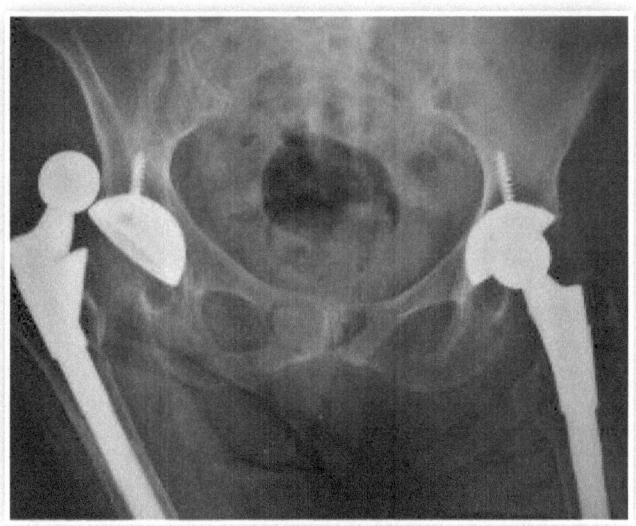
The right hip replacement has dislocated

Even more seriously, approximately two in 1000 patients undergoing a hip replacement will die in the process. The causes are usually of a cardiopulmonary nature and occur presumably because of factors outside the control of the treating team. Whilst all these complications are undesirable, they do not necessarily indicate negligence.

Conversely, if a patient suffers recurrent dislocation of a joint because the implants have been seriously malpositioned, a claim of negligence might be justified. Several tests may be necessary. The modified Bolam principle will be one. If it can be established that the surgical performance was substantially below that expected of a reasonably competent, appropriately educated hip replacement surgeon in Australia at that time, the test may be met. For evidence in proof of the absence of such a standard in a particular case, not all experts are willing to engage in cases of alleged medical negligence. Others are prepared to stand up and be counted. In such circumstances, I suggest that you engage an expert who has the experience, the wisdom and the courage to call it as it really is.

Oh, and be careful of interpersonal differences and TURF WARS!

LEAD ARTICLE

Dealing With The Difficult Plaintiff

A medicolegal consultation with an aggrieved injured plaintiff can be a very testing time for all involved. It can produce a heady mix of emotions including anger, resentment, frustration and fear.

It would be a very unwise medical expert who conducted it without recognising its potential for difficulty and conflict.

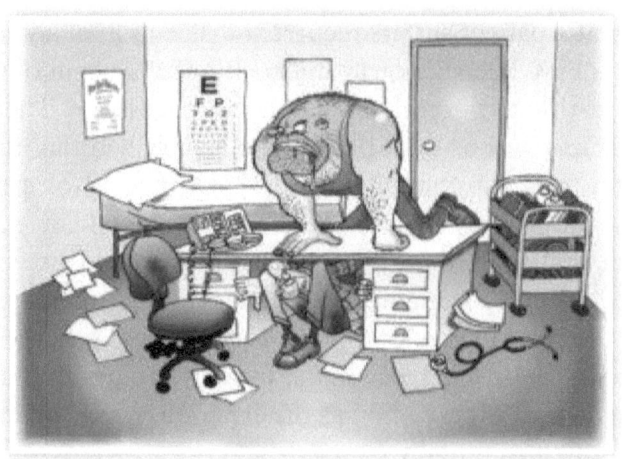

Grrrrrrr!

The process begins with my secretarial staff providing the plaintiff an easily digested three-page description of what will happen. I have written the document carefully and specifically. It avoids jargon and medical terminology. The plaintiff is invited to sit comfortably in my waiting room, and to read the material at leisure. It explains the basis of the consultation. I make it clear that I respect their position. It is also explained that I do not act for either the plaintiff's or the defendant's lawyers. My obligation is to provide an independent objective analysis without bias. I acknowledge my understanding of the stress that the person has endured and sympathise in general terms with the circumstance without confirming the presence or otherwise of any loss.

Allowing Time To Think

Prior to the consultation I also request the plaintiff completes a basic questionnaire. Questions such as date of birth, age, address, telephone number, employer, the date of the accident, type of accident, social and recreational interests and other such variables are canvassed. It gives the plaintiff an opportunity to focus upon their circumstance in private, and to provide answers without any pressure for a quick response. Even the simplest of questions can sometimes seem very difficult to respond to accurately during an oral inquiry in which the interrogator is waiting for an answer.

The Consultation

When the consultation begins, I welcome any support persons into my consulting room with the plaintiff and routinely apologise for making them wait (if that is the case). I acknowledge the difficulties associated with travel, parking and accessing my rooms. The purpose of this prelude is to put the person at ease, and to generate a rapport which will be non-confrontational and supportive. I avoid providing any commitment as to the outcome of the report.

During the first phase, I glean a history of the event and its affects. I also use a "90 second rule". This refers to allowing the plaintiff to tell their story in their own words at their own pace. Some are highly focused and specific and can accomplish the task in less than 90 seconds. Others may take 15 or 20 minutes! Whatever it takes, so be it. It means that the person feels content by having had some control of the consultation and being listened to. This is very important.

The Next Steps

At the end of that period, whatever it might be, I can then ask questions with more direction and elicit the details that are so important for the report.

This history phase is followed by a physical examination. Again, patients are often fearful and concerned that their discomfort may be heightened by the tests that are being performed. Generally, it is possible to perform a full physical examination without generating significant discomfort. Some tests can be a little unpleasant, but if performed carefully with skill, and accompanying solicitude, the discomfort is usually easily tolerated. A pre-emptive explanation goes a long way towards allaying any fears.

Occasionally, patients commence the procedure with overt aggression and a complete lack of co-operation. Rather than being offended by this, I regard it as a challenge. It is an opportunity to use some skill and empathy to defuse the negativity and convert it to co-operation and appreciation. The best accolade that I can receive is to be thanked by the departing plaintiff for the examination. Not all might be so grateful after reading the results of my objective analysis!

There are many features of an orthopaedic surgical career that provide great clinical enjoyment. From my perspective, however, very few reach the level that can be provided by a satisfactory medicolegal consultation, whatever its result.

CASE VIGNETTE

Do All Shoulder Injuries Require Surgical Intervention?

No.

Many patients over the age of forty years already have some intrinsic degenerative change within the soft tissue restraining structures around the shoulder joints. Those structures are collectively known as the rotator cuff and are formed by a concatenation of tendons passing between muscles around the shoulder joint and the upper end of the arm bone, and the surrounding capsule itself. That degenerative change is typically age-related, but it can be due to a variety of physical activities of a social, recreational, domestic or remunerative nature. Some are more susceptible to it than others. Many will be symptom-free, despite an abnormal MRI scan. Some from that asymptomatic group may still have partial or full thickness tears of a mild or even serious nature.

If an injury is superimposed upon these previously asymptomatic degenerative conditions, a symptom complex can become manifest. Typically, such patients will note a sudden onset of discomfort from a provocative manoeuvre, and will thereafter be plagued by pain, weakness, and often quite a significant restriction in range of movement.

Can Treatment Interfere With Litigation?

Yes.

Almost all such patients should initially be managed non-operatively. Over about a six-months period, many will improve considerably and may even return to their pre-accident asymptomatic state. This is despite the persistence of the underlying pathology.

Others may suffer with adhesive capsulitis or "frozen shoulder" during those six months. Its true cause is elusive. It is characterised by increasing pain and a concomitant reduction in movement. The pain typically reaches its zenith, and the range of motion diminishes to almost nothing. It prevails in a so-called plateau period for months, and then the whole process gradually reverses. The pain gradually diminishes, the range of motion begins to improve, and many will return to complete symptomatic normality. This frozen shoulder process may take as long as eighteen months. There is considerable debate about the wisdom of performing any operative procedure during that period. Some surgeons say that it should be well left alone until nature handles the matter as well as may be. Others believe that operative intervention can be of some assistance.

Whatever the correct answer, premature operative intervention can exacerbate the condition. Failed surgery may lead to revision surgery. Some patients may need to undergo a third bout of reconstruction. A subset of that group may even require a shoulder joint replacement.

When an observer casts his or her mind back to the original injury, and its natural history, some pity must be had for a patient who has been subjected to that course of multiple operations. Probably, it would have been better left well alone.

Who Should Pay?

The question then arises – who should be responsible for the outcome after that undesirable sequence of events? Should it be the original wrongdoer, or should the unwise orthopaedic surgeon share some of the responsibility for the total harm? This is a legal issue which is to be resolved by the Court according to the circumstances of the case. From a theoretical standpoint, both groups have contributed in some way. In practice; differentiating between the two can be very difficult. In my experience, it is usually the first defendant who carries the blame since medical negligence at law recognises the difficulty of medical decisions and imposes liability only in cases of serious departure from the medical norm.

GENERAL ADVICE

Derogatory Reports

The best medicolegal reports are those that are devoid of emotion and any shade of partisanship. A clear, non-polarised, objective report is a treasure. Unfortunately, some experts deviate from this standard.

The Shooting Gallery

This is characterised by the tendency for one reporter to lampoon another reporter to denigrate the latter's report.

This occurs most frequently in that section of a report dealing with impairments. Impairment guides are quite prescriptive (and proscriptive). Set processes are to be followed in calculating impairments, and any departure renders the assessment inaccurate and probably un-usable. However, not infrequently, the critical reporter's criticism is incorrect. Whilst the discredit cast upon the first reporter will eventually dissipate, it causes initial consternation within the legal profession. As experts' reports are exchanged and responses are received, the heat generated by the unjustified and ridiculing criticism will probably be reflected upon the critical one. He then also suffers.

This is not to suggest that inaccuracies should be left unidentified. Rather, a high level of professional courtesy is appropriate in exposing perceived errors. Critical observations can be courteously couched. After all, none of us can afford to live in our houses, which, in the end, are constructed entirely of glass.

LEAD ARTICLE

Plaintiffs' Docs and Defendants' Docs – Do They Exist?

Yes, I am afraid they do.

In fact, you all know who they are. One or two colleagues are "bleeding hearts" who accept at face value, and as fact, everything that plaintiffs say. They confirm losses far more than would be summated by their colleagues. These enormous differences in opinion usually result in our having to go to Court unnecessarily. Conversely, some reporters are particularly harsh, as though they have a universal suspicion against the truthfulness of an injured party who is seeking compensation. Neither extreme is acceptable. Objectivity, transparency, fairness, reproducibility, professional skill and common sense should form the basis of an expert report. A totally open mind in approaching each case, and reliance upon one's own expert knowledge to divine the facts that are reported, are essential.

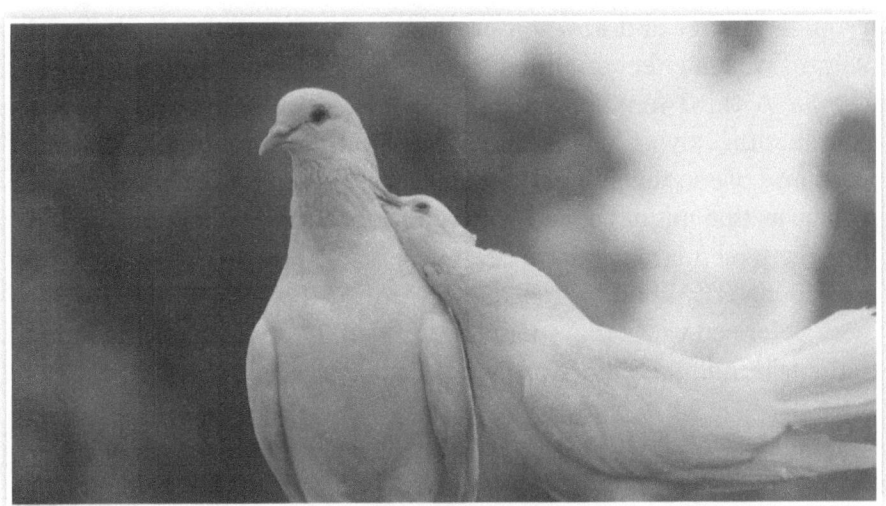

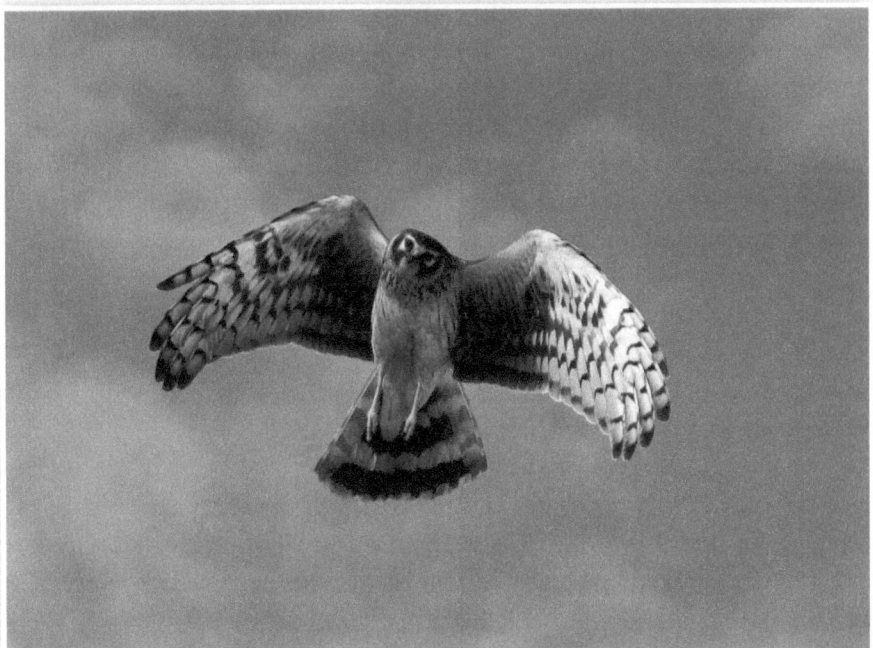

Hawks and Doves

I recall one of my older colleagues, now retired, who believed that every plaintiff was "bunging it on". He was of the view that almost regardless of the impairment that had been sustained, the plaintiff could still be an Olympian. Another colleague seemed to believe that no matter how trivial the injury and how minor the impairment or the disability, the plaintiff was in effect qualified to receive a Disability Support Pension forever. A third famous colleague, whilst being subjected to cross-examination, joyously suggested that "well he measured 15% and I measured 5% so the judge'll just make it 10% and we can all go home". As true as that might be, had both reporters come in accurately at 10%, then the trial might not have been necessary. The time, the stress and the expense could all have been avoided. At the front of the line, it is these polarised views that should be avoided. Despite their presentation to the tribunal, mediators or judges usually see through the mist.

It is understandable why a plaintiff's lawyer may seek a softer, more supportive opinion, whilst one who is acting for a defendant's indemnity insurer may wish a harder line. They are doing their duty to investigate the matter thoroughly and to present to the Court the most persuasive evidence available. As a means of avoiding the dangers of unreliable reports that might lead to a large increase in the costs of an unnecessary contest, there is a trend for the lawyers for both plaintiffs and defendants to co-fund a single objective, middle-of-the-road report from an expert whose balance is recognized and respected. This trend is to be applauded and encouraged.

CASE VIGNETTE

Overreaction And Inconsistency

Not all patients are 'ridgy-didge'. Not all patients are as badly affected as they have one believe. Not all presentations to an expert can be explained in purely medical terms. Some patients overreact, behave inconsistently, embellish their condition, or may even be true malingerers. Not every case is as it might seem.

Differentiating between real and contrived presentations can be difficult and requires experience and skill to counter. Expressing an opinion on the matter requires care and sensitivity.

There are no precise tests which can accurately and routinely differentiate between the real and the asserted, but there are some tests which may indicate any inconsistency and/or overreaction. Useful tests include the application of different forces, at different times, in different locations during an examination. Sometimes a plaintiff may perform identical functions in different situations differently. Huffing, puffing, moaning and groaning are also noteworthy.

Their interpretation should be carried out judiciously. If they are positive, they should be identified and explained in detail in the report. A courteous way of referring to the differential may be in the phrase "The presentation does not conform with any medical condition with which I am familiar". Referring to the claimant as a liar is to be condemned.

GENERAL ADVICE

Who Should Provide Medicolegal Reports?

Experts.

That sounds like a glib response to the question but it implies some special truth. It is a special calling.

Medicolegal reporting is a subspecialty, in its own right. For many years it was viewed by aged and retiring clinicians as an avenue to supplement income into twilight years. As their clinical practice ran down, and in the absence of healthy superannuation portfolios, some experienced a financial pinch after retirement. They would drift into medicolegal reporting, relying upon decades of clinical experience, and in the process, impose untested and sometimes erratic views upon the Courts.

That is not to say that all retiring clinicians have behaved so. Some have been extremely valuable and accurate.

The point, however, is that age and clinical experience alone are not sufficient to guarantee excellence in this field. There is no substitute for experience, and a good reporter will have experience within that arena. It is not a recreation or a casual money-spinner for the amateur. A true professional in the field will be a regular attender at medicolegal conferences, subscribe to medicolegal journals and be open to constructive criticism and advice from all members of both professions.

The best are those who enjoy providing such reports, engage in continuous medicolegal education, and are open to the ever-expanding horizon of this specialty.

LEAD ARTICLE

Should Medicolegal Reports Be Solicited From A Treating Doctor?

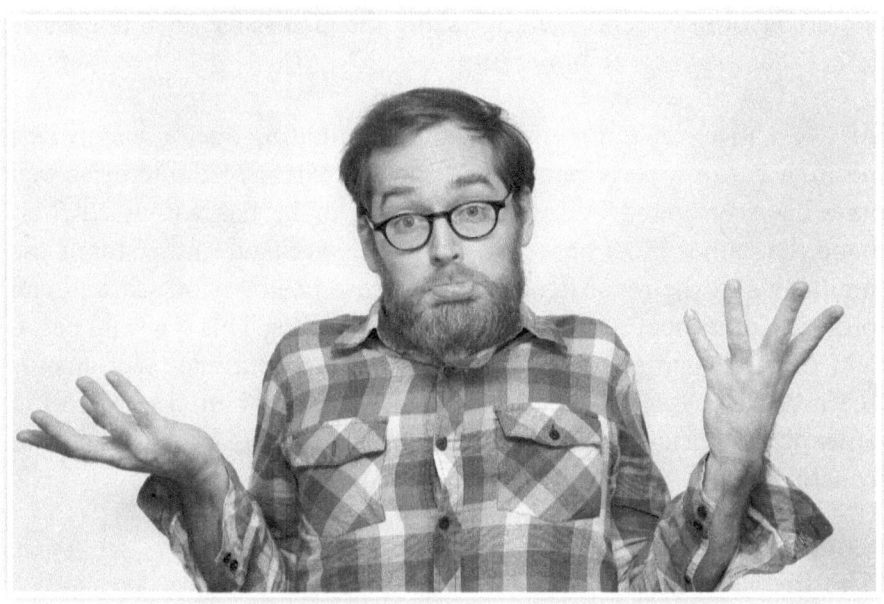

Reports are sometimes solicited for tendering in Court from a doctor who has been intimately involved in the management of a plaintiff's injuries, and from those to whom the patient has been referred for specialist treatment. The reports from these practitioners are tendered as evidence of the history of the injuries, and their treatment and progress. They are usually vital to the admissibility of reports of expert witnesses, since they form the basis of the opinions formed. The expert reports may not otherwise be admissible.

The concern with sole reliance on reports of treating doctors is that an unconscious bias might exist. It could form through the close relationships developed during treatment of the subject injuries, and, perhaps, similar bonds built up through years of medical consultations. The assessment could lack objectivity.

There are many issues to consider. It would be reasonable to expect that a treating doctor may have some considerable sympathy for a patient. It is also possible that there may have been some complications because of the treatment protocol. Worse still, it may be that the doctor did not perform as well as may be desired. In any or all these instances, the clinician may be tempted, consciously or subconsciously, to provide a more favourable report, embellishing the losses sustained and those losses that may accrue in the future.

An alternative viewpoint might be that the treating doctor is truly best positioned to properly understand the full extent of the injuries that have been sustained by the plaintiff. She or he has witnessed first-hand the pathological havoc that has been wreaked, understands the limitations of the reconstructions that have been performed and can provide a more accurate perspective on prognosis. This is a valid point, and so the essential report from a treating practitioner will answer the needs to which it refers. Nonetheless, an additional report from an expert reporter who is at arm's length from the patient has plain benefits.

The Professional In Action

A third dimension of influential factors is relevant to the overall professionalism of the reporter. It requires an ability to be divorced from any emotional link to the assessment and to engage in true, unencumbered objectivity. Recognition of any potential for conflict of interest is mandatory. However, what if the injury spectrum under report forms part of a highly specialised niche in medicine where few other qualified reporters are available?

I do not have a strong view on this matter one way or the other. There are strengths and weaknesses in securing reports from treating doctors only, though the weaknesses are cured by the simple means of obtaining reports from both sources. There are also problems in securing a report from a non-treating "expert" who is poorly equipped to provide medico-legal reports.

In the final analysis, it is probably best to assess each case as it comes and make a value judgement on an individual basis.

Yet Another Dimension

Many years ago, I had a 20-year-old male patient with a hip injury. He suffered with a condition known as avascular necrosis of the femoral head. Part of the ball on the upper end of his thigh bone died and was destined to collapse. He was far too young for a joint replacement, so I performed a fresh osteochondral transplant. This involved retrieving a compatible segment from the femoral head of a cadaveric donor and transplanting it into the patient's hip. It was novel surgery at the time. Prior to his claim being tested at trial some years later, I assessed him for the purposes of quantifying his impairment and disability. He told me his hip was excellent and essentially pain free. My opinion was based in part on his perception of clinical success. Understandably, the insurer was delighted.

During cross examination by his Counsel, it was put to me that really his condition was far less good. He'd given me a rosier picture of reality because of an unspoken fear that I might want to operate again!! Well .. what could I say. In this case, the treating doctor was not of much value.

CASE VIGNETTE

Scarring And Other Things

Patients sometimes sustain lacerations resulting in scars. Others require operative intervention which also results in some scarring. Scars will vary in their severity, extent and cosmetic importance.

Chapter 8 in the AMA 5 Guides deals specifically with scarring and the principles of assessment of scars. Table 8-2 on page 178 is instructive. Five classes of scarring are described. At the minor end, Class I yields a loss of between 0 and 9% of whole person function. At the other end of the extreme, Class V yields a loss of between 85% and 95% of it. Most patients will be within Class I. A loss of between 0% and 9% can therefore be added to their combined losses for the purpose of quantifying general damages.

It is also possible that scars may be of such cosmetic importance that plastic surgical revision is indicated. Additional costs will be involved and these should be quantified prior to resolution of the claim.

Some workers' injury compensation insurers have their own unique assessment methodologies. These should be consulted if they are relevant.

GENERAL ADVICE

Do X-rays Lie?

The problem does not reside with the x-rays. Instead, potentially it is with the viewer, and in this context, that refers to the expert reporter who is interpreting them.

There is an old saying that the clinical circumstance cannot be better than the worst x-ray image reveals. Not all radiographs will depict an underlying problem. Conversely, if a problem is depicted, it is real.

Another interesting concept is present in the folklore that patients with exceedingly severe degenerative changes on an x-ray can be completely unaware of the condition at a clinical level. The cervical spine is a classic location. Patients can have extremely severe degeneration at all levels from the base of the skull down to the upper thorax. The disc spaces may be almost completely obliterated, large spurs may have formed, the end plates could be extremely sclerotic (appearing white on the film) and osteophytes have protruded out and almost completely obliterated the intervertebral foraminae (the canals through which the exiting nerve roots are obliged to pass). Despite the severity of these findings, a plaintiff may claim to have been completely asymptomatic, completely unaware of any problem in the neck prior to the subject accident which is the basis of the claim.

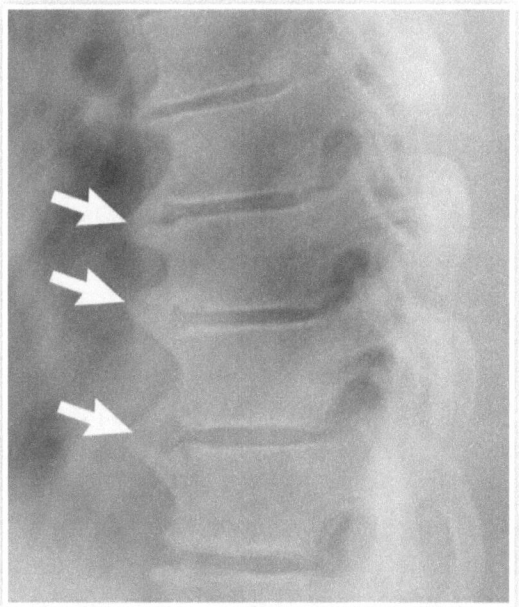

The arrows point to large degenerative spurs which have bridged anteriorly

The only time I ever experience this circumstance is in association with the Court room. Perhaps we should "never say never" in medicine, but I haven't otherwise seen a patient with such radiographic evidence to be completely asymptomatic.

It would be worthwhile to be wary of this presentation if you encounter it.

10

LEAD ARTICLE

Interesting Cases

As I look back over 40 years of medico-legal reporting, I estimate that I have produced more than 10,000 reports. This is a conservative estimate, and I am confident the number is significantly greater.

Plaintiffs of all shapes and sizes, of various genders and predilections, and from all walks of life and circumstance, have presented, with extraordinary variation in degree of impairment and disability. Prior to the introduction of the "5% rule", cervical spinal injuries predominated. (This "5% rule" is peculiar to Queensland, Australia. If the quantified whole person impairment is less than 5% for any claim, under the personal injuries legislation it is not allowed to proceed.) My understanding is that most plaintiffs with a cervical spinal injury that exceeds that 5% limit can be guaranteed a minimum gross payout in the order of AUD$60,000. Costs will obviously chew up a fair part of that award, but the endeavour still appears to be worthwhile. Many lawyers will conduct the claim on a "no win, no fee" basis.

I also see patients who have suffered with injuries in road traffic accidents, workplace accidents or in domestic incidents. Occasionally, they present with particularly interesting problems.

What A Surprise!

One afternoon, in a consultation with a lady in her sixties from interstate who had sustained a cervical spinal injury, we went through her history taking and examination phases without difficulty. At the end of a 40-minute consultation, I was ready to assist her to the door. Rather than stand as I had expected, she remained seated, impassive for a few moments and then wept. For no special reason, she told me an unrelated story. She had me believe (and I do believe) that I was the first person with whom she had ever really discussed it during her adult life. She had been married twice, had three children, yet she had never shared this memory.

Her Story

She grew up in a small country town in western Victoria. She believes that her memories probably dated back to the age of three years. She could recall regularly sitting on the top step of three timber steps at the front of her home in the mornings and the afternoons, gazing out at the road, the nearby houses and nothing in particular. Every morning without fail, a man who lived several hundred metres up a gentle hill to the left of her home would drive down the slope, heading to work. He would invariably slow his vehicle as he approached her home and, though never stopping, he would gaze in her direction. This would be repeated in reverse in the afternoon as he was driving home.

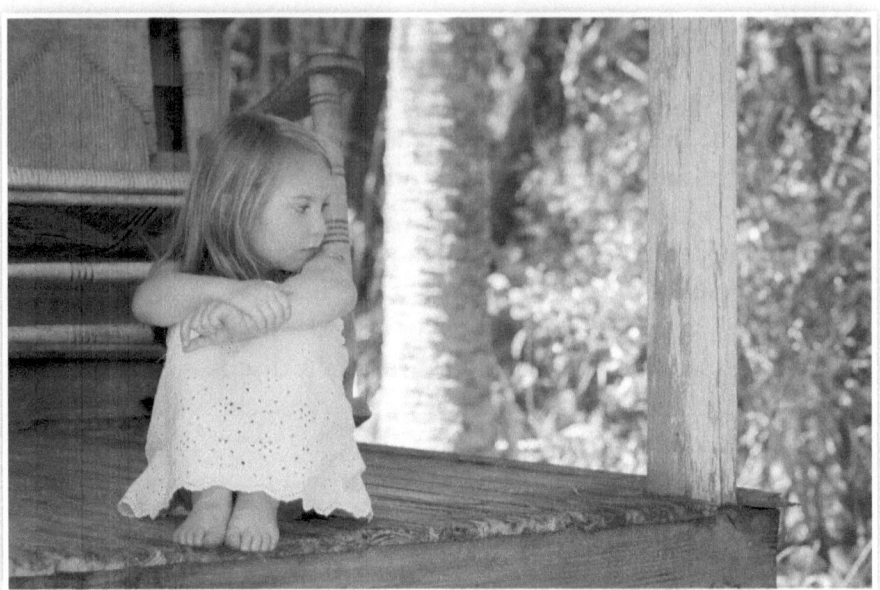

A Feeling Of Dread

She was not sure how long this pattern had persisted, but thought that it was probably several years. She was about six years old when one afternoon, instead of simply slowing and continuing past, the man stopped his vehicle adjacent to the grassy verge. He alighted from his car, walked through the front gate and up the steps beside her. He entered her home without addressing her.

From the shadowy interior she heard the muffled voices of him talking to her parents. Some short time later (it may even have been an hour), he came out of the house onto its verandah, accompanied by her parents. The man was carrying a small cardboard suitcase which, she later learned, contained her clothes. After a brief conversation with her parents, she left her home, boarded the car with the man, and was driven that several hundred metres up the gentle slope of the hill to his home. He then took his own daughter, with a suitcase filled with his daughter's clothes, back to my medicolegal patient's former home.

It had transpired that both girls had been born in the same hospital on the same day. There had been a mix-up in the nursery, with the result that each was taken home with the wrong parents. In those three, four, five or six years, as the man drove past the patient's home, he realized that the girl whom he saw sitting on the front steps was his true biological daughter. The child who was living with him belonged in that other home.

Over the intervening five decades or so, the patient's life was generally quite miserable. Although her biological father was loving and affectionate, he died when she was only eleven. Her biological mother was most distressed by this re-arrangement. Unaware of the mix-up, she had grown very attached to her non-biological daughter and was extremely resentful of the exchange that her husband had effected.

The patient had some contact with the other girl over the next decade or two and it appeared that although her relocation was uncomfortable at first, her biological parents formed a warm and special bond with their own daughter.

My medicolegal patient had lived all these years without ever having revealed her story to others. By the completion of the tale, she was sobbing uncontrollably in my consulting room. I, too, was deeply moved.

I remember the afternoon well. My waiting room was full. I was running late. I had heard a most moving narrative, and there was absolutely nothing I could do. I did comfort her and uttered soothing words but given the distress that she had suffered and the duration for which it had continued, my contribution was nothing but a pittance.

Her medicolegal claim was the least of her worries. This event caused a change in my life.

CASE VIGNETTE

Some Foot Injuries Are More Severe Than They First Appear

The foot has three components: (a) the hindfoot with the calcaneus (heel bone) and the talus (the ankle bone), (b) the midfoot with the tarsals and the bases of the metatarsals, and (c) the forefoot with the metatarsals and the toes.

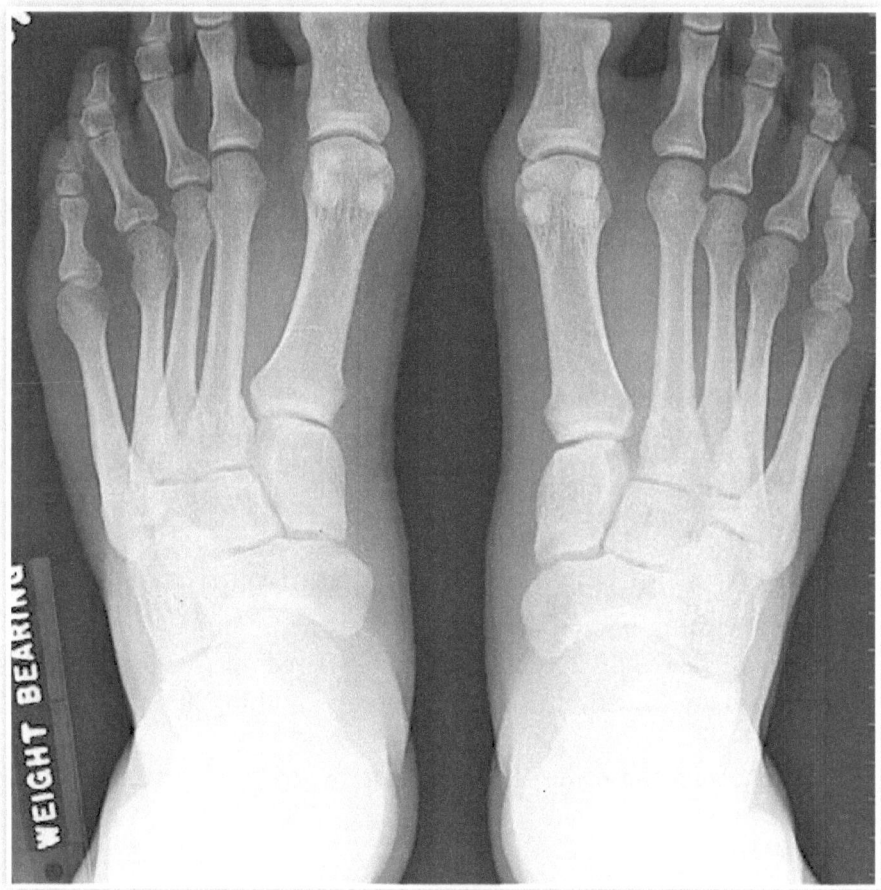

Hindfoot and forefoot injuries are usually obvious. Midfoot injuries, however, can be mistakenly overlooked. Its combination of joints is sometimes known as the "Lisfranc" joint. This description refers loosely to the junction between the talus and the calcaneus behind, and the cuneiforms and the cuboid in front. The latter (the cuneiforms and the cuboid) also articulate with the bases of the first to fifth metatarsals inclusive.

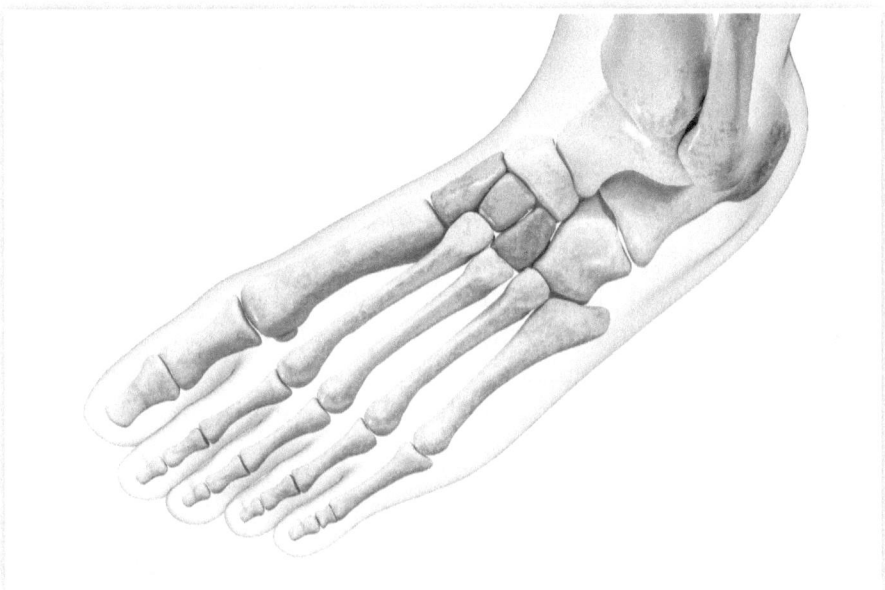

This constellation of joints is of low range but imparts an ability for the midfoot to circumduct, that is, an ability to go upwards and downwards, inwards and outwards, and rotate. The shoulder circumducts too, but its range of motion is vastly greater than that in the midfoot.

Twisting or crushing injuries can give rise to midfoot fractures with or without associated dislocations. They may be difficult to detect clinically and with plane radiographs. Computerised scans are usually clearer, and MRI scan examinations can also more accurately delineate the extent of the disruption. Technetium bone scans can sometimes be of use.

Many midfoot injuries of the fracture plus dislocation variety are missed. Healing takes place with the joints in deranged positions and with ligaments stretched, contracted or distorted.

Osteoarthritis Supervenes.

The midfoot's performance thereafter is permanently diminished. Afflicted patients will often present with stiffness, pain and midfoot swelling. They have difficulty wearing footwear, standing for prolonged periods, ascending or descending steps and slopes and negotiating uneven terrain. If the plaintiff is a labourer, considerable remunerative losses may ensue.

From an expert opinion perspective, the AMA 5 Guides are not particularly useful. This injury is not described in specific terms. References are made to an increase or decrease in the height of the arch of the midfoot and allowances are also made for x-ray appearances consistent with post-traumatic osteoarthritis. It is possible, however, that the plaintiff may have quite severe symptoms, marked limitations in ambulatory capacity and a severe interruption in lifestyle without those obvious features. Chapter 17 of the AMA 5 Guides may yield very little in the way of determining functional impairment though the disability can be quite large. It is imperative that the expert reporter understands these concepts and explains them in detail rather than by prompting by the Court.

After all, how could the Court be expected to know? Defence counsel, even if advised of it by their own expert, is not likely, and is not required, to raise it if the plaintiff's expert has not done so. Whilst there may be an excellent understanding of the legal intricacies of the plaintiff's case, the Court cannot act on the possibility that an underprepared or ill-equipped expert will be sufficiently wise to provide direction and advice.

This is another reason to choose medical experts carefully!

GENERAL ADVICE

Are Literature Reviews Useful In Negligence Claims?

Don't expect to read about any tricks here. There are none.

Instead, there is a strong averment that scrutiny of all the records and radiographs, separation of complications from under-performance, a careful analysis of the current state and the garnering of at least one objective expert report should be the mainstay of the process.

Contemporary literature reviews are useful, though not all clinicians regularly read them. Trainees or those about to sit their Fellowship examination would be the most avid visitors to scientific literature. That interest is often maintained for a year or two, or maybe a decade, but thereafter, many medical experts "fly by the seat of their pants" and only occasionally add to their current literature intake. If they work in a hospital setting, many attend journal clubs and "Grand Rounds". Their knowledge of most current concepts is casually gathered from specialty conferences and workshops where nothing more than the surface is often scratched.

Experts producing a report might suitably cite the literature. It is important that the publication does not postdate the sentinel event and is freely and generally available. Review articles are preferred to those that delve into minutiae or esoteric matters.

It would be wise for instructing solicitors to seek copies of the papers that have been referred to and to attempt to make their own judgement in consultation with their expert. An external opinion on the publications could be valuable. Not all are as relevant as might be claimed. In fact, some quoted publications are not relevant, or worse, confirm the opposite. Be vigilant.

11

LEAD ARTICLE

How Complex Can Complex Matters Get?

It is obviously a question involving many normative issues and factors of degree. How deep is the ocean? How long is a piece of string? When, for a child, will the car journey end? (Except 'soon'!)

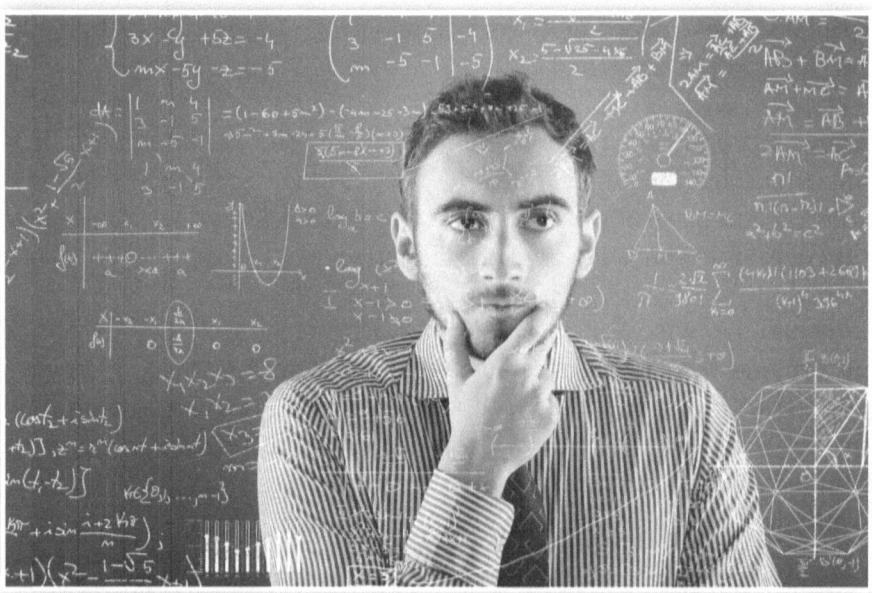

Causation is a topic in point. Sometimes, the answer is relatively easy. The penetration of a chainsaw through a thigh, or an axe into the back of the head, a person's being crushed beneath a steamroller or being given a live and detonated hand grenade; all of which can be expected to give rise to serious and obvious injuries and are usually clear circumstances of causal connection between the action and consequent injury. Conversely, the dropping of a pin in the presence of one who suffers the onset of deafness a week later would raise serious issues for a claim for compensation based on the noise caused. The difficulty of attribution of causation may arise for some patients who may suffer quite serious conditions of essentially unknown cause or aetiology.

A relatively young woman whose first pregnancy was complicated by quite severe osteoporosis involving one hip (you will read more about this condition later) had several significant co-morbidities, some of which could be associated with osteoporosis. Usually, osteoporosis is of a global nature and not linked specifically with a single focus. She suffered a fracture of the hip near the end of her pregnancy and had a joint replacement. Complications ensued, and the outcome was far from desirable.

Her litigation against her treating clinician alleged inaccuracy of an initial diagnosis, a delay in making the correct diagnosis, and delay in instituting a proper therapeutic regimen. The quality of the treatment was also questioned. All in all, an unhappy sequence.

In the absence of a specific identifiable cause, it was difficult to find a breach in the diagnostic or therapeutic processes. Although the outcome was obviously adverse, in the absence of that link between the duty of care and the care that was provided, on the one hand, and the harm, on the other, the claim based on negligence was understandably in difficulty.

Measuring residual impairment can also be extremely difficult in some forms of injury. Reference is usually made to authorities such as the American Medical Association publication, "Guides to the Evaluation of Permanent Impairment" (5th Edition) or similar publications. They are no more than just guides. They often rely heavily upon the measurement of joint movement, or lack thereof. The extent of the manifestations of these functional defects can vary from day to day or even hour to hour. On a very good day, a patient may have a permanent impairment of only 4%, but on a bad day, it could be three times higher. This is despite its having reached maximal medical improvement.

The possible presence of such variation makes the translation of impairment to general activity very difficult and often unwise. The difficulty can also be found in social, recreational, domestic and remunerative competence. It becomes extremely complex to determine the true state of a plaintiff and to advise the Court accordingly.

The solution to complexities is not avoidance. Rather, it is imperative that all options are considered, identified and enunciated. A best fit is chosen, and the reasons for preference are explained clearly so that they can be tested and, if justified, be demonstrated to be so.

As openness increases and clarity becomes more obvious, so does complexity diminish. Experts who can distil, and explain, and justify complex matters to their essence are of most use to litigants and the Court.

Remember, impairments and disabilities are different concepts.

CASE VIGNETTE

Hand Injuries Can Be Difficult To Assess

Next to the brain and the eye, the hand is one of the most complex human anatomical structures. The precise placement of its bones and the astonishing array of its tendons, ligaments, nerves and blood vessels forms an anatomical unit capable of truly extraordinary pursuits.

It can remove a small bead from a nostril or wield a sledgehammer to smash a large rock. The wrist, the hand, the thumb and the lesser digits combine in a most magnificent way. Mathematical formulae have been used to describe the synchronous movements involved in dexterous activities. *Google* 'Fibonacci' sometime.

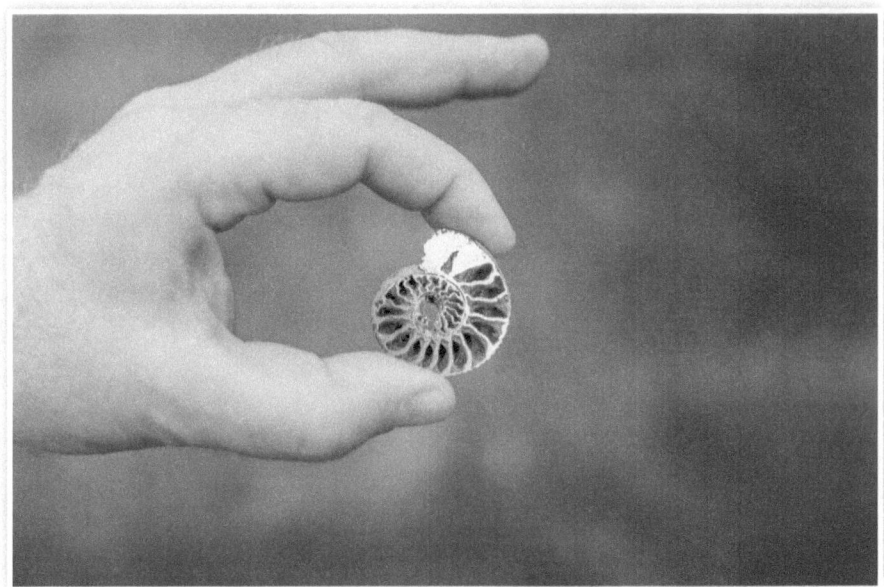

A natural Fibonacci sequence

Unsurprisingly, therefore, serious hand injuries can have major adverse consequences. Assessing them requires special skill by the expert reporter, and the consultations can take considerable time.

The AMA 5 Guides (Chapter 16 in particular) provide precise instructions. Every joint is to be assessed individually, every tendon and nerve function has been considered. Variations on radiographs will have been described and functional components can be considered either in isolation or in concert.

For the assessment of practical impairment to the patient's activity, dominance or non-dominance of the limb is important, as are other factors, such as the prior education, training and work experience. A right-handed barrister who loses his left hand in a rock-climbing accident will obviously be unhappy at the outcome but will not be so severely disabled as a concert pianist. Remember though, they may exhibit the same impairment.

A medicolegal assessment of hand injuries is among the most complex tasks that an orthopaedic surgeon can be asked to perform.

GENERAL ADVICE

Which Cases Should You Accept?

Obviously, this will vary according to your persuasion, but it is desirable that a practitioner accept references without preference. This generates experience of all extremes, the middle ground, and cases in between. Rather than being exposed to just plaintiff or defence perspectives, the expert develops balance and circumspection. The potential for bias is reduced.

In any case, it is of considerable importance to the respective parties that a report accurately reflects the true position. This facilitates taking the most suitable course in the further pursuit of action. It should avoid finding at the end of a costly trial that submissions failed because of defective evidence.

It may not be a question whether the plaintiff was injured but whether the consequences were as serious as claimed. If a defendant has made a 'without prejudice' offer of an amount that corresponds with or exceeds the later award by the Court, the plaintiff may be ordered to pay the defendant's costs of the action as well.

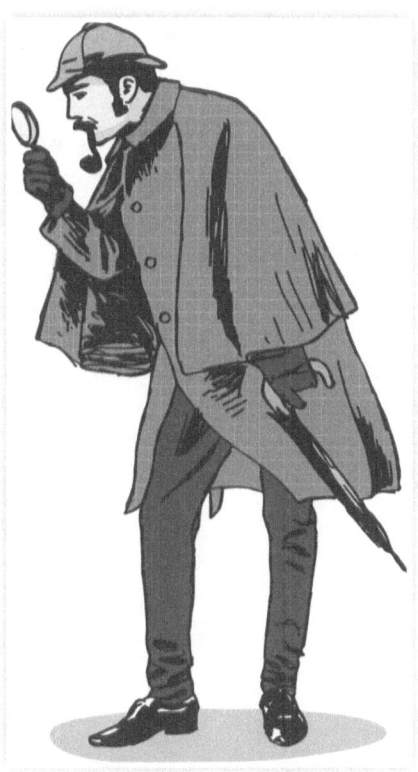

If the defendant is wrongly advised, the defendant may unsuccessfully defend the action, particularly as to the quantum of damages, and be liable for all costs when, if having been properly advised, it would have negotiated a settlement and avoided most of the costs.

In an assessment by the plaintiff's own expert, there are a few simple steps that should be taken. The first relates to consideration of the likelihood that an injury to the extent claimed has really occurred and whether there is some measurable impairment or disability. If the claim sounds trivial, it may well be trivial. If there is a cogent history of what appears to have been a major insult, then real incapacities and disabilities may have the benefit of consistency.

Another step relates to the magnitude of the impact of the injury on the social, recreational, domestic and remunerative prospects for the claimant. Although significant scarring has occurred, it may be confined to a part of the torso which is routinely covered by clothing and not normally visible. It would therefore be of less gravity than severe and multiple facial scarring on a young woman.

The amount of an award may depend in part on the plaintiff's perceived honesty and presentation. Inconsistency, overreaction and embellishment are sometimes quickly apparent. Then, it is probable that the medicolegal reporter will have antennae which are receptive to it.

Similar considerations apply to the task of the defendant's reporter. If there is a history of likely genuine injury, a well-documented sequence of medical events necessitating considerable therapeutic intervention, and a cogent medicolegal report attesting to the veracity of the claim, contesting it may plainly be a losing battle. There could be an exception - that the claim is excessive and unjustifiable – and it is the task of the reporter to assess whether it is so, and to discover and reveal its flaw. In general, however, pedantic obstinacy over tiny increments could be wasteful for all involved.

What About Recurrent Claims?

At the other end of the spectrum for the defendant lawyer's attention is the recidivist claimant. As many as eight, ten or even a dozen previous claims over the previous few years should raise some suspicions about verity. This is not to say that a person could not be so unfortunate, but as the number of claims increases, so does the chance that there is a motive for deception for personal gain.

In essence it is a wise precaution to assess it all carefully, consider all options and make a balanced, cautious and realistic value judgement.

A final step which could be very valuable is to call your favourite medicolegal reporter and ask for some *ad hoc* unofficial discussion as an aid to clearing the mind. A fifteen-minute conversation could save considerable fruitless expense.

LEAD ARTICLE

How Useful Are Prior Medical Records?

A sage answer is "vital", but there are some obvious exceptions.

For a competent assessment of a functional loss or quantification of an impairment, and for the task of attributing that loss, or a component of it, to a compensable event, it is important to be aware of any loss that may have predated the subject injury. Apportionment in this way is sometimes overlooked and can lead to unrealistic expectations and wasteful litigation.

Caution should be exercised since past medical records can be erroneous or misleading. Many years ago, I appeared as an expert witness for the defence in a provincial District Court. The plaintiff had allegedly injured his back in a lifting incident whilst working. As we walked up the steps of the District Court, the defence barrister informed me he had read somewhere in the plaintiff's past medical history that he had sustained some form of back injury. I accepted this at face value and inquired no further.

Whilst adducing my evidence, the barrister mentioned this prior history of back problems and asked whether that, rather than the accident in question, could have been responsible for his current state. I foolishly agreed. Foolish for several reasons. First, I had not taken a history from the plaintiff about the event that had allegedly occurred prior to the subject accident. Nor had I read the notations to which the barrister had referred me earlier, and I had no idea of the significance of this antecedent problem.

The cross-examining barrister appeared to be about as naïve as I was and did not raise it. My downfall was brought about by the judge himself. At the conclusion of the cross examination, he asked me for more detail about this past medical history and how it could influence the opinion that I had expressed in my report. He produced the documents in question, and they revealed that the patient had previously suffered with a mild episode of coccydynia. This condition affects the coccyx and not specifically the lower lumbar spine. Apparently, it had arisen "out of the blue" and without any precipitating traumatic event. There was no prior history of back problems and my unwise apportionment of blame was exposed for its worthlessness. This was a most embarrassing moment and one of my many lessons.

In another and much larger claim, in which I was not involved, the claimant was a young woman dancer at the Gold Coast who suffered an injury of some significance to a foot. Specialist orthopaedic and treating general practitioner evidence expressed the opinion that as a result, she would never be able to engage in that career again, which was true. As the general practitioner was called to give evidence, his record cards as to attendances and treatment of the injury under his care were tendered. It was the trial judge's scanning of the cards for the period prior to the injury that was revelatory. For some period prior to the relevant injury, she had consulted the general practitioner for a developing condition of her foot brought on by her professional dancing activity. When gently taken further by the judge, the general practitioner acknowledged unequivocally that the condition would have naturally deteriorated in any case and would soon totally prevent her from dancing. None of this had been mentioned in the medical reports that had been tendered to the Court.

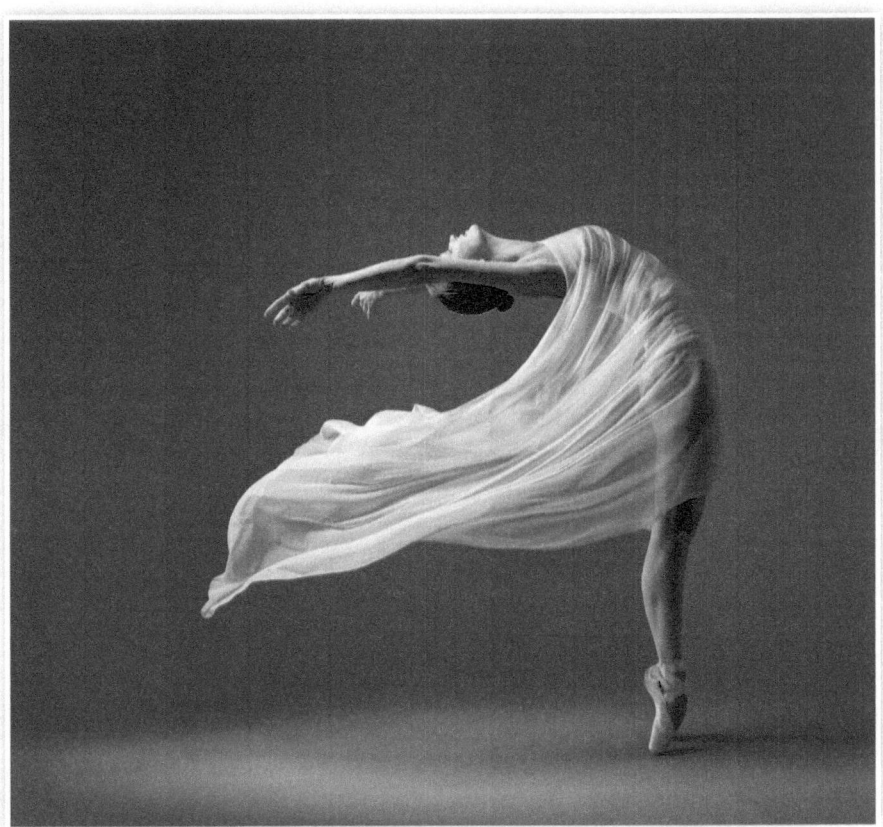

There had been other evidence that she was extremely talented, and would be successful in Hollywood, thereby earning a very considerable fortune, which had been the basis of the large claim. At the judge's suggestion, the parties sought an adjournment. The claim soon settled, presumably at a much-reduced sum.

Whilst past medical history is of vital importance, it deserves to be carefully scrutinised. It may be of some value in the final analysis, or it may be totally unrelated. If it be related and of significance in the determination and is deliberately ignored and not revealed by a reporter, it would be discreditable.

CASE VIGNETTE

When There Is Nothing To Be Found, Is It Possible Nothing Has Happened?

Although injured parties can almost always clearly explain an event, it is sometimes more difficult to relate that description to the claimed effects. Relatively trivial accidents can result in quite debilitating pathologies. Generally, there is a direct and visible relationship between the magnitude of the applied forces and the physical outcome. It will not be surprising that medicolegal reporters are sometimes confronted with an obvious mismatch. Injuries such as a simple tap on the shoulder have been claimed to have caused a broad spectrum of suffering in the neck, the back, the hips, the knees and even in the feet. If there has been little or no injury, it is more likely than not that little or nothing has happened.

Strange things do happen, but they are rare. There may be some benefit in accepting injury spectra just outside the norm as genuine and compensable, but if no injury has been sustained, there should be no compensation. The best expert reporters will call it as they see it ... and explain why.

Advocates for the claimant have a duty to maximize the claim, but in this, common sense must have its place. Those acting for the defendant are not blind and nor is the medicolegal reporter.

GENERAL ADVICE

Where Does Medicolegal Experience Come From?

The answer is obvious. From many and various places, really.

From a medical perspective, competence is directly proportional to experience. That is not to say that they are equal, but as medicolegal reporters age and gain experience, they refine their process and diminish or even eliminate obvious errors, commissions or omissions. There is an adage that "Good medicolegal reporting comes from experience: experience comes from bad medicolegal reporting". It would be a very unusual medical practitioner who engages in medicolegal reporting without a few mistakes. It is hoped the reporter will have learned from that experience.

From the legal perspective, experience is also important. Whilst the legal aspects of managing a claim are outside a medical expert's domain, so, too, is a deep understanding of anatomy, physiology and pathology for many lawyers. It is sometimes surprising how much medicine some senior legal practitioners know and understand, but there will always be some voids and deficits. Several relatively easily digested texts deal with medicolegal issues, and explain some of the nuances of injury, impairment and disability. Another useful port of call is to telephone your friendly medicolegal consultant. This type of dialogue assists both sides. There is no property in a witness. There is no reason why these frank discussions cannot occur. Provided the rules of evidence are obeyed, considerable mutual assistance can be gleaned.

LEAD ARTICLE

How Do You Give Plaintiffs Bad News?

Whilst this lead article is directed principally at lawyers who are acting for plaintiffs, it may also be of some assistance to defendant lawyers. I refer particularly to the difficulty associated with advising a client about an expert report that it far less supportive of the client's case than had been hoped for.

Some Background

Plaintiffs have typically been injured in workplace, motor vehicle or domestic incidents. They have suffered some form of insult, have been exposed to pain and discomfort, have experienced social dislocation and feel genuinely aggrieved. Some may perceive an irreversible adverse change to their lifestyles.

Though all of these may be felt, they are not always deserving of compensation in our current medicolegal system. Consider a patient who already had a long list of prior serious comorbidities and was functioning sub-optimally. There may have been severe lumbar spinal disease, an arthritic hip or knee joint, neck pain or discomfort, or adverse outcomes from surgery.

The subject accident related to the claim may have further injured those sites, but difficulty arises because the effects are either immeasurable or invisible. Moreover, the added insult may have made little, if any, difference to the natural history of the antecedent condition.

An Example

A plaintiff in his mid-fifties was working as a steel fabricator. He'd suffered with a severely arthritic hip joint for some years. His pain would already have caused him difficulty. It would have been noted whilst getting into and out of his car for going to and from work. He could barely have bent over at his bench to pick up a piece of steel from the floor and would have constantly been looking forward to the next meal break so that he could rest. It was already destined to affect his future remunerative prospects markedly and adversely.

One day, in a road traffic accident on his journey to work, he sustained a fracture of his thigh bone just below this affected hip joint. It required hospitalisation, operative intervention and six months absence from his work. The orthopaedic intervention was so effective that the fracture united in a perfect position and without any specific adverse sequelae.

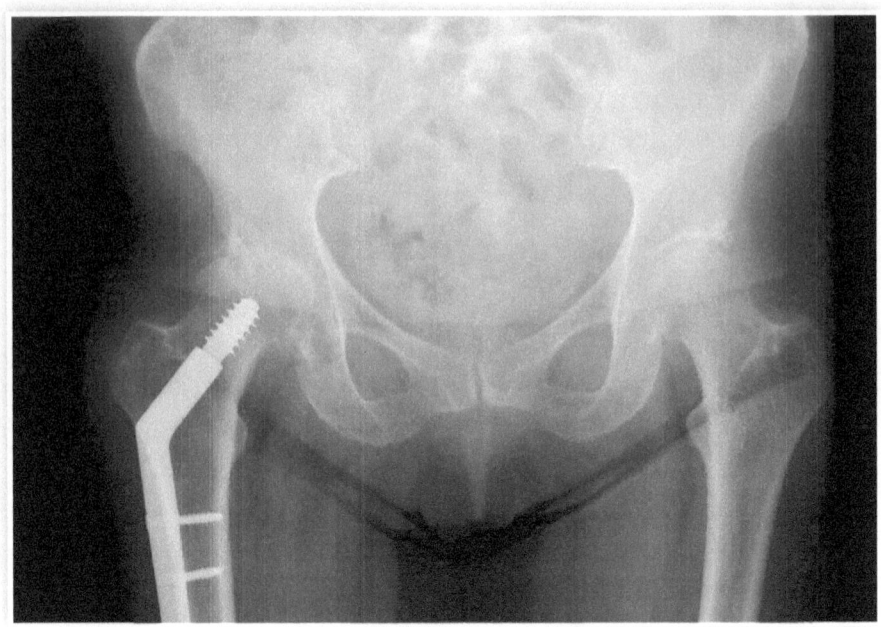

The metal devices have stabilised the fracture below the arthritic joint

Under normal circumstances, he would have made a perfect recovery. As it eventuated, his recovery was far from perfect because of the preexisting hip arthritis. He might understandably believe that the road traffic accident had contributed to his hip problem, foreshortened his working life, exposed him to considerable remunerative losses. and diminished his ability to engage in a broad spectrum of activities of daily living.

Unfortunately, whilst his beliefs might be genuine, they are not necessarily right. The accident has made very little difference other than necessitating the fracture surgery, imposing the prolonged hospitalisation, and causing temporary added pain and suffering. It did not measurably alter his hip arthritis. His outcome is representative of the prior arthritis, not the accident-related injury. His compensation in damages will be limited to only those added features.

Alternatives Exist

The preceding example must be distinguished from the position where the resulting pain, suffering and disability from the accident are much greater than the prior condition caused, or would have caused. His condition was altered by the accident. His clinical condition had been (permanently) aggravated and heightened. His physical competence was additionally diminished. That the prior condition was a contributing factor, to the extent of the consequences of the accident, was of lesser importance, for a wrongdoer must take the victim as he finds him.

So, how do you give this bad news (to the plaintiff or the defendant)? It is not easy. One way is to allow the party to read the expert medical report without making any emotional or derogatory comments. The same approach is desirable in relation to the contents of an adverse report which is provided to whichever party commissions it. Every word of it should be expected to be made public, and the litigant has the right to know what has been written. If the reporter's thought process has been cogent, objective and fair, the party's reading of the report may go some way towards assuaging any anger and frustration that might otherwise be experienced.

From a lawyers' perspective, it might also be best for the report to be open and transparent, as well as caring and comforting. In the final analysis, it is best to know the truth from the outset. As painful as it might be, it could save tens of thousands of dollars and years of anguish with fruitless litigation.

CASE VIGNETTE

The Scars Were All On The Inside.

Catherine was a 45-year-old mother of three young children, happily married and working full-time as a primary school teacher in a provincial centre.

She was driving on a country road in a 100km/hour zone and approaching a T-intersection. An oncoming Ford sedan, travelling in the opposite direction, was stationary on the highway, waiting to turn right at the T-junction while Catherine was proceeding straight through.

As she approached, the Ford sedan was struck from the rear by a following truck and was pushed into a collision with Catherine's vehicle. Its driver was fatally injured, instantly. Catherine survived but sustained a plethora of very severe injuries. Both collar bones (clavicles) and nine ribs in the left chest wall were fractured, and she had fractures in the right chest wall. Her central sternal segment was "floating" and both lungs were punctured. She had a massive haematoma around her heart, and like Steve Irwin (the crocodile hunter), she was suffering from cardiac tamponade. This is a situation that occurs when blood is being pumped out of the heart through a rent in its muscular wall but the surrounding pericardium (a non-expansile sheath) remains intact. The pressure that builds up inside this pericardial sac compresses the heart and gradually but inexorably stops its ventricular muscle from pumping. Untreated, death is inevitable. Having been retrieved promptly, transported without delay, and subjected to immediate open-heart surgery, Catherine survived, but only just.

Both clavicular fractures and chest wall injuries united satisfactorily. Most clavicular fractures heal without residual sequelae and it is very uncommon for rib fractures to cause long-term pain. Both of her lungs reinflated, and, apart from the longitudinal scar down her anterior chest wall, there was very little visible evidence that she had suffered those injuries.

Her Claim

Six years after the accident, there was very little to see apart from the scar. Both shoulders were functioning satisfactorily, the claviculae were pain-free and her chest wall also expanded relatively normally. The AMA 5 Guides gave her a 0% impairment of whole person function in purely orthopaedic terms. (There was a small component for the chest wall scar under Chapter 8).

She was never the same again, but, surprisingly, for a reason unconnected with her own injuries. Despite the absence of any form of contributory negligence on her part, she felt responsible for the other driver's death. No amount of counselling could dissuade her. The inconsolable anguish wreaked irreversible damage upon her marriage, her family and her friendship group. She did not return to work, she isolated herself from her previously close community, and she clearly expressed the view that she felt her life was not worth living. It was a most tragic case.

There was no permanent or serious orthopaedic feature that provided mileage for her claim. All her "scars were internal". Suffice to say, she did have significant social, emotional and remunerative loss claims. This was left to the psychiatrists.

GENERAL ADVICE

Too Soon, Too Far

There is a question as to when it is appropriate to have a plaintiff examined for medicolegal purposes. When does the patient reach Maximal Medical Improvement? When is the condition caused by the accident stable and stationary?

Maximal Medical Improvement (MMI) is an important term. It denotes a state, and a time, when the plaintiff is unlikely to become any better following a compensable injury. Some recover fully. Others never. Many reach a peak and then begin to deteriorate. The medical expert is retained to comment upon this concept of MMI, and whether future related costs may eventuate. With this assistance, to the extent that it is accepted, the Court awards compensation.

So When?

There is no easy answer, although some yardsticks are available. For example, patients suffering from musculoligamentous strain injuries of the cervical spine (the "whiplash" injuries .. the term I abhor), can still show signs of gradual but significant improvement for up to 18 months after the accident. Measuring an impairment or quantifying any loss prior to that time could be premature. This will be of special relevance to defence lawyers since their client may be pressured to pay prematurely and excessively. A large sum paid on settlement may later seem to have been mistakenly generous if that plaintiff eventually returns to complete symptomatic normality.

Conversely, there are some injuries which declare themselves in their entirety immediately. Irreversible quadriplegia with complete transection of the cervical spinal cord will not recover. Although marvellous advances are being made with stem cell therapies, no current or future therapy is envisaged for such a devastating lesion. Rather than wait for months or years for signs of relevant improvement, it may be kinder to all involved to assess and settle early.

The Medical Expert's Role

The medicolegal reporter has an obligation in this respect. Through no fault of anyone, some solicitors may refer their client for assessment and report sooner than would normally be desirable. For example, a cervical spinal musculoligamentous injury may be sent for an examination and report ten months after the accident. The expert should not provide an opinion then because Maximal Medical Improvement has not been reached and a quantum impairment assessment is not reasonably possible.

An alternative is to advise that MMI has not yet been reached but, if the trial is in progress, by way of assistance, and given the natural history of the condition exhibited by the plaintiff, the reporter could provide some advice to the Court. For example, that the claimant may exhibit features consistent with Diagnosis Related Estimate Category

II in Chapter 15 of the AMA 5 Guides. This would yield a loss of between 5% and 8% of whole person function. The plaintiff may still be suffering with quite marked symptoms with non-verifiable radicular signs and reach that 8% threshold. Although there are indications of continuing gradual improvement, the magnitude of the injury may cause the medicolegal reporter to consider that a return to normality is unlikely. Since some further improvement was probable, the eventual loss may reduce to something in the order of 5% or 6% of whole person function.

This type of opinion, expressed transparently and with full explanation, could be of great assistance to both sides of the legal table. Despite the assessment's being slightly premature, a more informed discussion could take place at mediation or settlement negotiations, to the benefit of all involved in that time, money and stress may have been saved.

No two medicolegal assessments by reporters are the same, but there are common themes. This is one of them. It would be useful if all medicolegal experts engaged at this level.

14

LEAD ARTICLE

The Paradigm Of Assessment Of Future Economic Loss Is Changing

Most personal injury claims have a component for future economic loss. Injured plaintiffs typically will lose wages at some presently indeterminate time or times after an award. Even if they have sufficient paid sick leave or income protection insurance policies to span this unexpected gap, their use of it may diminish its value, contingently upon the appearance of other demands for their invocation. Additionally the ability of the plaintiff to return to former activities may be seriously compromised, with a need to be confined to lesser duties attracting lesser pay.

It is useful to the process to offer a spectrum of future employment for the plaintiff to the Court for it to consider. Typically, those roles can be subdivided into sedentary, semi sedentary or laborious in nature. Over the last 30 years or so, I suspect that I have placed thousands of call centre operators, car park attendants, gate attendants, telemarketers and waitresses. All those jobs have been filled!

In this second quarter of this 21st century, occupational demands are changing dramatically. Those who are relatively unskilled yet desirous of significant incomes are attracted to mining and resources industries. It is not uncommon for an unskilled or semi-skilled person to earn more than AUD $250,000 per year as a fly in-fly out miner.

Many of those tasks plainly require physical competence and strength. Duties include the operation of large and potentially dangerous machinery, lifting heavy objects, working in confined spaces and manipulating heavy tools. Only a fortunate few in these fields will have more sedentary duties in an office or be restricted to a kitchen or a store warehouse. With the vagaries of the international export market, it is probable that those enjoying these jobs will find that they will not last forever.

In this new era, plaintiffs with an education will usually be operating regularly with computers. Some could be trained as programmers, whilst others will still be required to enter data. Telecommunication roles and opportunities in the auditory and visual arts will also appear. Consultancies and adviserships may expand in a world of nuance. Artificial intelligence starts here. Those without an education or formal trade skills or qualifications will find the future much more challenging. Sales jobs with incomes based on commissions will proliferate. Share-ride driving could be an option for part-time employment, and a small subset of plaintiffs will opt out of society and live "off the grid", on the public purse.

So What Do We Do?

In essence, our ability to cope with the employment needs of our injured population is not keeping pace with the movement of future remunerative demands and opportunities. This will lead to an increased burden upon our already strained systems of insurance. Premiums will rise, social service demands will climb, and litigation in this personal injury sphere is likely to become more common.

Do you have any solutions? Astronauts maybe?

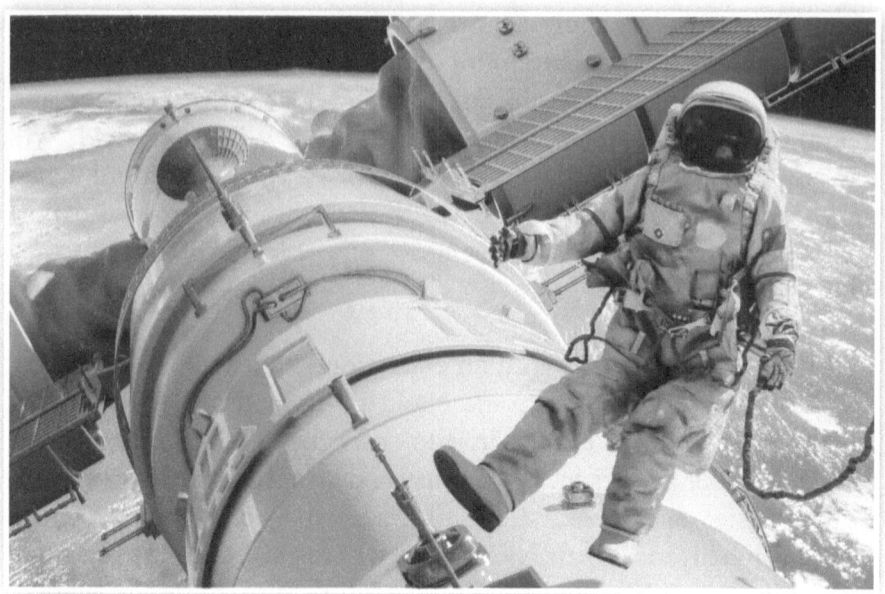

CASE VIGNETTE

Are MRI Scan Examinations Important?

Sometimes!

There is no substitute for taking a full history and performing a thorough physical examination. A good clinician can usually make a correct diagnosis in 85% or more cases with just those two useful tools. Plane radiographs will increase the accuracy to the region of 92%. Of difficult diagnoses, the remaining 8% can usually be secured with additional investigations, such as CT scans, MRI scans, bone scans, PET scans and blood tests.

MRI scan examinations are most useful in analysing soft tissue injuries, but they can be used to assess bony or skeletal injuries too.

A patient in his fifties had suffered a knee injury. Even though he was adamant that this knee had formerly been completely asymptomatic, plane radiographs performed within a few days of the injury revealed a significant abnormality. He had an avascular region of bone necrosis in the medial femoral condyle. This was a discrete volume of dead bone forming part of the lower end of the thigh bone (the femur) and would have been present prior to the injury. It is possible, however, that he was completely unaware of it at a clinical level. Thorough scrutiny of his prior medical records failed to reveal any prior complaints. His Counsel could then reasonably submit that the benefit of the doubt lay with him.

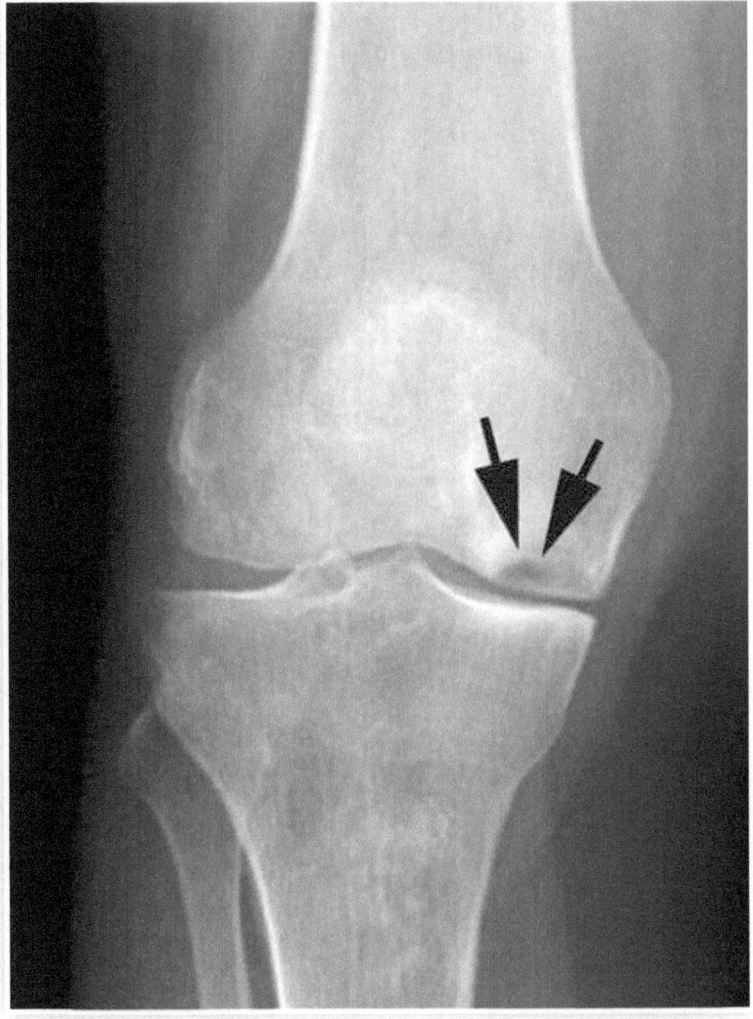

The arrows show the affected region in the medial femoral condyle

Can MRI scans depict lesions that plane x-rays miss?

They can, and that is what happened in that case. The defence argued that the subject injury had simply unmasked this condition and had not really caused any damage or harm. Fortuitously, the claimant had an MRI scan examination just three weeks after the accident. Not only did the scan show these old changes of avascular necrosis involving the medial femoral condyle, but it also showed oedema in the bone and the soft tissues in that region. Oedema refers to interstitial fluid in the tissues (outside cells and blood vessels) and is indicative of a recent injury. So extensive was the oedema in the soft tissues and associated bone that it was reasonable to assume that quite considerable forces had been applied to the joint at the time of the subject injury. At least some of his presentation was due to the injury.

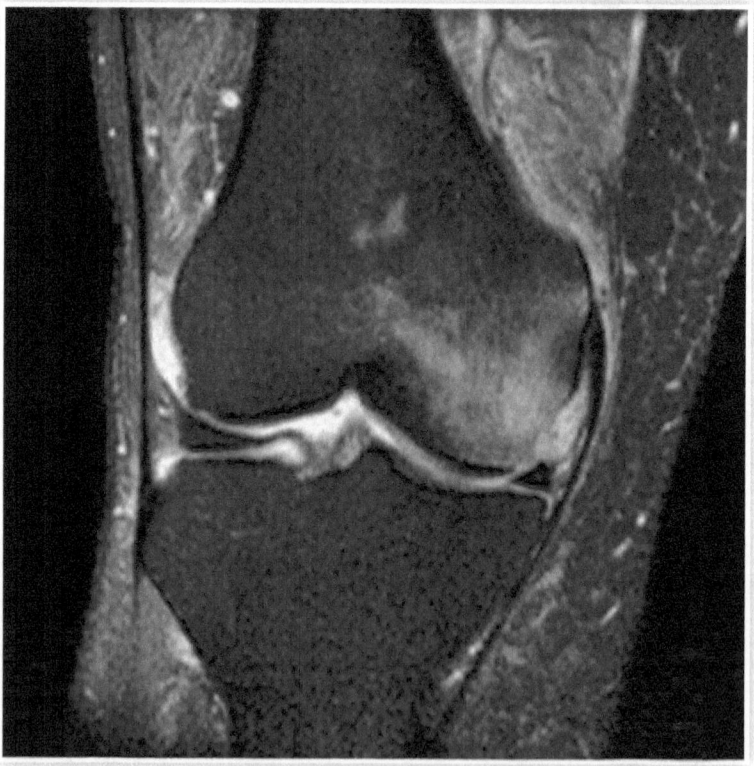

The MRI scan shows oedema (whiteness) in that same region

This became of considerable importance. Although he had been asymptomatic prior to the injury and it could be reasonable to assume that he may have continued to be asymptomatic for some considerable time, his clinical course was altered by the injury. Furthermore, within six months, he had undergone a partial knee replacement. Unfortunately, that intervention failed and within thirteen months, he had to undergo a total knee replacement. It, too, was not particularly successful and, given the fact that he was still in his fifties, it was more likely than not that he would eventually require a revision of that total knee replacement.

He had therefore gone from being completely asymptomatic to being subjected to two major operations which still left him encumbered.

His claim was successful, and the quantum of his award was thought by the defendant to be extremely generous. That may have been the case, but had it not been for the MRI scan examination findings, it is possible that he would have received much less than he was justly entitled to.

The effect of the MRI scan examination appeared to be pivotal.

GENERAL ADVICE

Should A Solicitor Accompany A Client To A Medicolegal Examination?

That is a matter for the relevant parties and seems to have no prima facie significance. Most solicitors are content to allow their clients to attend examinations without legal support. In more than 10,000 medicolegal examinations over the last three or four decades, I received only a few such requests. I always acceded. It would be most imprudent for a solicitor to endeavour to manipulate the examination or coerce an expert, but some plaintiffs have great difficulty focusing their attention on specific questions and may give erroneous responses. In suitable circumstances, the presence of an interpreter or a friend, relative or support person may be desirable or even essential. Occasionally the whole family attends!! I rustle up extra chairs.

Can A Lawyer's Attendance Assist?

When assessing a claim, a medical expert is interested in the past medical history, since it can be of vital importance. It could, as to a final clinical outcome, influence a potential apportionment of blame to any injuries sustained. A patient's account of prior medical history may not always be accurate, even without dishonesty. A claimant with a back problem following an injury may be forgetful or disinclined, in anxiety of appearing to be complaining of trivia, to mention that he or she had experienced some vague aches and pains long previously. Clinical records subsequently produced in evidence and disclosing that such attendances had been made on a general practitioner or a physiotherapist would contradict the claimant's denial and could diminish the credibility of the remainder of the history provided by that party.

An advising solicitor may recognise that this detail is of little or no significance to the assessment as almost all persons experience some back pain sometimes. Whereas many are content to resolve it by means of a paracetamol tablet or two and calmly bear it, others are less robust and may too quickly seek the advice of a general practitioner or a physiotherapist. Those consultations do not necessarily imply any major structural problem referable to the lumbar spine. Whatever the problem had been, it may have settled completely. It may have no relevance to the subject claim following the more recent injury. But the damage to the client's credibility overall by a failure to disclose the matter may be seriously disproportionate. In these circumstances, an attending solicitor with his or her client may avoid an injustice by giving suitable ethical advice.

As the law dealing with personal injuries continues to expand, solicitors may more readily attend formal medicolegal examinations and reviews with their clients. That would have my support.

LEAD ARTICLE

Can Lower Limb Surgeons Comment Upon All Orthopaedic Matters?

Possibly.

Orthopaedic surgeons in Australia and New Zealand, with Australasian qualifications from our College and Association, undergo an exceedingly rigorous programme before Fellowship is conferred. All facets of orthopaedic surgery are covered in the training programme over an extended period and, whilst subspecialisation is both recognised and encouraged, the basic elements of orthopaedic surgery are required to be entrenched and never forgotten. These principles apply in most North American States, Canada, the United Kingdom, many European countries and South Africa.

What Is Expected Of Them?

I have concentrated solely on hip and knee surgery for about two decades. Prior to that, I spent a similar period performing lumbar spinal surgery, upper limb surgery and dealing with maladies of the foot and ankle. Even now, I still attend general orthopaedic continuing professional development programmes in national and international fora, and hospital morbidity and mortality meetings which include all subspecialties. Refresher courses, updates and new horizons are canvassed and covered. Most also subscribe to international journals which concentrate not only on our subspecialty interests, but also contain articles of generic orthopaedic value.

This medicolegal orthopaedic specialist is trained in the relevant authoritative texts used to assess impairments. The American Medical Association publication entitled "Guides to the Evaluation of Permanent Impairment" (5th Edition) is the most common reference, but similar others are available. All have chapters dealing with all regions of the musculoskeletal system. Accreditation as an Independent Medical Examiner requires competence in all systems and regions.

Therefore, it is not necessary to send an upper limb problem to an upper limb surgeon or a spinal problem to a spinal surgeon. That is not to say that selective referrals are discouraged or disallowed. Instead, it means that a medico-legal expert should act within his or her competence as an analytical reporter, an objective observer and a credible Court performer. It is unnecessary to seek a subspecialty qualification in the anatomical region that has been adversely affected. However, it is important to choose the medicolegal reporter wisely. Reputation, skill, objectivity and clarity are arguably more important than a distinct clinical interest or flavour.

CASE VIGNETTE

A Simple Stumble - A Lifetime Of Misery

A 45-year-old male sustained a knee injury while leaving work at 5:45pm in winter when it was already dark. He was leaving a donga on a work site in a geographically remote location. There was only one down step from the donga to the uneven ground, but for some unknown reason, he tripped and fell. He did not roll to the ground but took the impetus of all his weight on his right foot while his knee joint was partially bent. His torso twisted to the right. He experienced immediate pain in the right knee.

He was taken to a local hospital, where he spent the night comforted with analgesics and elevation, and was then referred to a regional centre for further assessment. He had sustained fractures involving the upper end of his shin bone (the tibia) and both sides of the tibia that contributed to the knee joint (the tibial plateaux). The fractures were displaced and the joint surface was no longer pristine and smooth. The treating surgeons opened the fractures, reduced the fragments as best they could and used metal plates and screws with some biosynthetic bone graft to reconstruct the upper end of the tibia. Valiant as the efforts were, a successful anatomical reconstruction could not be achieved. Over the next 20 months, he was treated with braces, physiotherapy, crutch ambulation, analgesic ingestion and several programmes of rehabilitation.

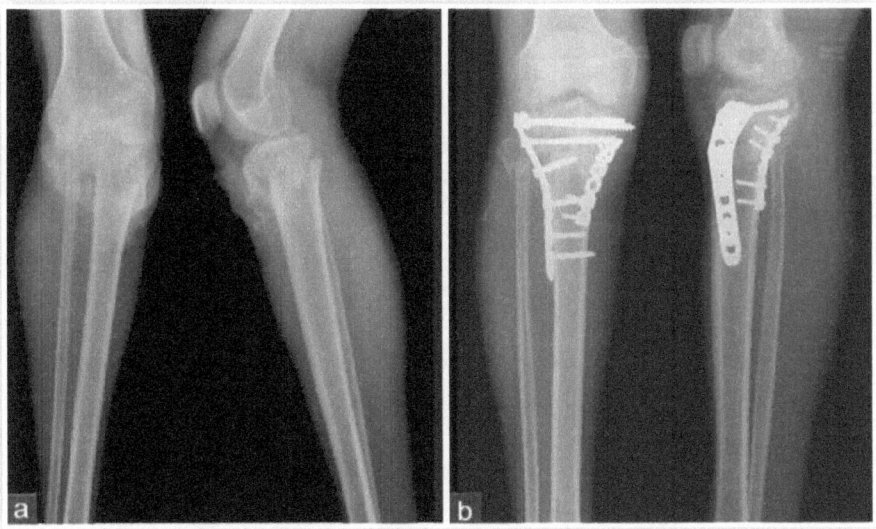

Preoperative (a) and postoperative (b) images

As nature would have it, the fractures healed, but the joint surface was no longer congruous. In addition, surrounding soft tissues had been damaged quite severely. Though the ligaments remained intact, the enveloping capsule became adherent to the lower thigh bone and upper shin bone so that the knee joint became stiff, painful and swollen.

Clinical and radiographic examinations confirmed that this knee joint was not retrievable. The patient was likely to require a total knee replacement within the next couple of years. He would be in his late forties. When performed in patients in their sixties, the arthroplasty or artificial joint has a survivorship of approximately 90% at 20 years. Stated differently, only 0.5% of these joints fail annually for those two subsequent decades. Failure is defined as the joint requiring revision or a second replacement.

The results of knee replacements in younger men are not quite as good and his expected failure rate could be twice that. By the time he is 70, he has a 40% chance of that joint's requiring a revision knee replacement. The primary replacement would have cost in the order of AUD$50,000. The revision would cost in the order of AUD$60,000 in current values.

Apart from his knee, this patient was in excellent health. There is no reason to believe that he may not live until his mid-eighties or even longer. His father lived to 101 and his mother, though dying in her early seventies, had been fatally injured in a road traffic accident. Baring that misfortune, and based on her medical history, it is probable that she would have lived until her late nineties or even beyond. This patient's genetics were such that he could also live at least that long.

That raised the spectre of a 15%-20% chance of his requiring a re-revision, or a second revision, knee replacement. Costs in the order of AUD$70,000 may have been incurred.

Added to the complexities of these surgeries is always the risk of complications. Arteries or nerves may be damaged. Deep venous thromboses may form and emboli may travel to the lungs. He may have a stroke or even a debilitating cardiac event. The infection rate for the primary arthroplasty is only about 0.6%, but with revisions, the infection rate may double, treble, or even quadruple.

Such a simple fall, therefore, can precipitate a very unpleasant further forty, fifty or even sixty years. Unless the reporting expert is aware of these scenarios, any plaintiff is at risk of being severely under-done at the time of settlement. Choose the expert wisely, not only to detect the spurious complaints, but also to beware of the possible future ramifications.

GENERAL ADVICE

When To Appeal A Workers' Insurance Tribunal Decision

Most jurisdictions have a statutory authority charged with ensuring the health and welfare of workers. When faced with a claim for assistance, it behoves it to confirm the genuineness of the claim. After all, it is the public purse that is being opened.

These custodians of that treasure usually request an Independent Medical Examination (IME) prior to forwarding a claim to a Tribunal for determination. Claimants can be disadvantaged by referral to an incorrect specialty or to an expert lacking the appropriate competence to report.

Injured workers have the option of having an external second opinion. There have been many occasions where this has proved to be a worthwhile exercise and though it adds additional cost to the process, it is desirable if doubt is ever present. If the second opinion agrees with the first, so be it, and the doubt is resolved. Alternatively, if they are diametrically opposed, one is incorrect, and a third opinion may be necessary.

Objectivity, fairness, and distance from any emotion that attends a workers' compensation claim are important. If an injured worker reasonably feels hard done by, a second opinion is a very useful comfort.

LEAD ARTICLE

Keeping It Simple

Litigation is complex enough. Having an expert who further muddies the waters must border on the intolerable.

Though some plaintiffs experience a constellation of complex, almost overwhelming injuries, it is possible to distil the outcome to a single simply stated essence. This is the key to professional medicolegal reporting.

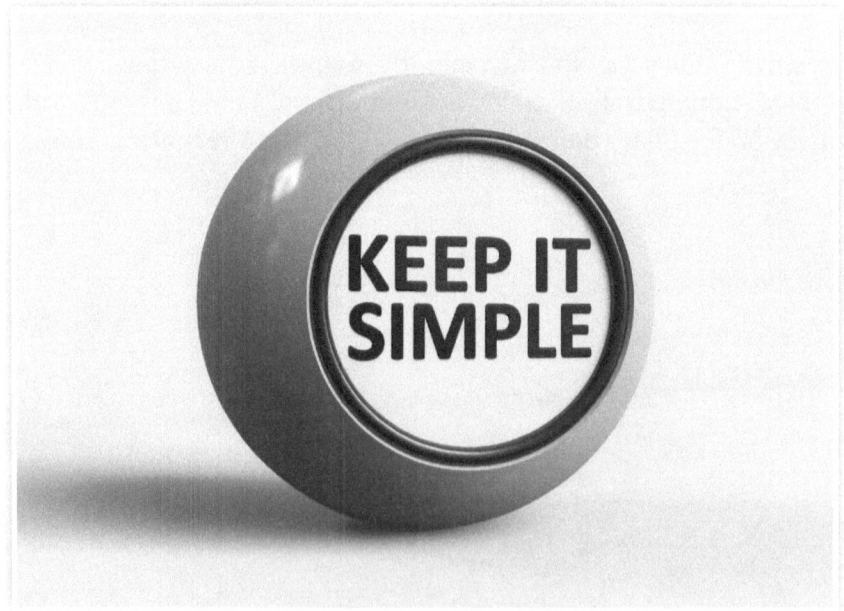

The analysis may be compared to a funnel with layers of filters. At its top, the diameter is wide and all facets of the relevant circumstances can be poured in at random. As they move down through the filters towards the outlet, so can the matters be sequentially refined, summarised and collated.

By the time a report emanates through the spout, all its readers should be presented with a clear, concise and cogent distillate. All components of this complex process should be combined to provide a very clear analysis of causation, impairment, disability and future losses.

Such clarity comes from not only the written word, but also from a visual appreciation of the form in which the report is presented. Report layout matters! It can be tedious and tiresome to read a ten-page typed report, single spaced, and with untidy margins and no headings, let alone sub-headings. All the relevant information may be contained in it, but the form resists its efficient extraction. Gleaned details may be clouded in jargon, ambiguous in thought, and bordering on the useless to anyone other than the author.

It should be the aim of the medicolegal expert to keep it simple, while every factor, every facet and every nuance should be included. This can be accomplished with succinctness and clarity of thought. It should be crafted in such a way that, so far as it can validly go, there is no doubt about the injury, its detail, and its effects on the plaintiff.

When expressing an opinion, alternative views should be clearly, fairly and fully canvassed, with an explanation of the author's reasons for differing and preferring the opinion advanced.

CASE VIGNETTE

It was 1979

A 16-year-old girl was brought into the Accident and Emergency Department on Saturday afternoon having been involved in a relatively high-speed motorcycle accident with her boyfriend. She was a pillion passenger, and they were in remote bushland. The cyclist lost control and they struck a large gum tree.

She had not lost consciousness but was unable to stand. She lay unattended for more than 90 minutes before being retrieved and transported to hospital. On assessment, she was found to be suffering with extreme knee pain. A clinical examination that included radiographic investigations failed to reveal any obvious problem in the region of the knee joint. Oral analgesics were prescribed, and she was discharged into the care of her parents. Her father remembered carrying her out to the car.

In the early hours of the Sunday morning, the girl was still in great pain, distressed and dissatisfied. Her parents represented to the emergency department with her.

On a review of the x-rays that had been taken the previous day, it was observed that although the knee joint appeared normal, the radiograph itself was suspicious. See if you can identify the problem.

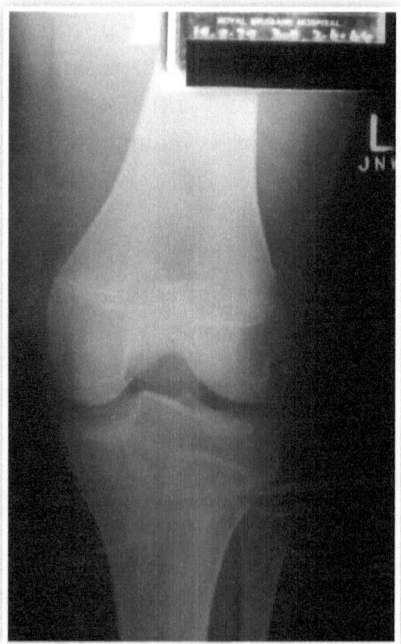

Can you spot the problem?

At its top, just to the left of the name plate, there is something protruding downwards and to the left. On the x-rays that were taken on her re-presentation the following morning (depicted below), it is demonstrated that there was a transverse fracture of the femur (the thigh bone) with considerable overlap. The lower end of the upper segment was protruding down and laterally beside the name plate. Unfortunately, the x-ray taken on that Saturday did not extend high enough.

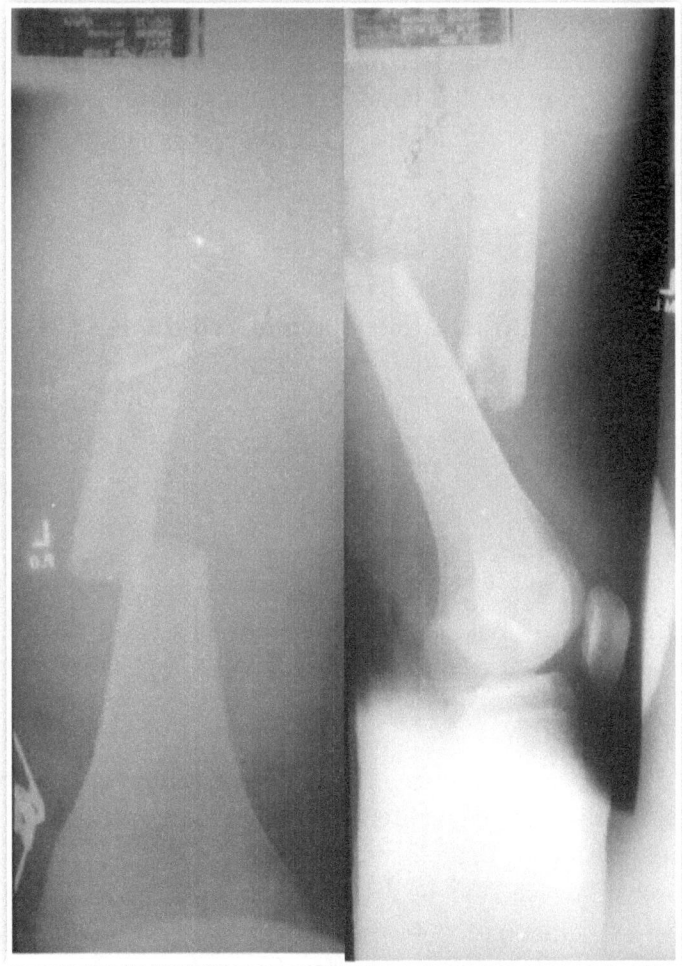

See it now?

This transverse fracture of the thigh bone was untreated for upwards of 20 hours without adequate analgesia, crutches or splintage. Her parents were obliged to deal with her bodily functions in her bed overnight and on the next morning. As the bones protruded into the soft tissues in her thigh, she would have experienced extreme pain. All this was the result of inadequate physical and radiographic examinations. Even a cursory examination of the thigh would have identified this complete fracture of the femur.

It was a very valuable lesson. There but for the grace of God go I. Good orthopaedic surgery comes from experience and experience comes from bad orthopaedic surgery. It is best if experience comes from the mistakes of others and not those of oneself. This was a poignant experience.

GENERAL ADVICE

Dealing With Administrative Appeals Tribunals (AAT)

This is not a commentary on dealing with the AAT: that is not my function. Instead these are my observations of a process which might be flawed.

The general legal concept of liability appears to a layperson to be a little loose or flexible. Conversely, the rules under Personal Injury Protection Acts and Civil Liability Acts seem relatively straightforward, and causation is well described. The waters appear to be murkier within the AAT.

Defence Force personnel present a particular challenge because some of the claims result from activities that occurred twenty, thirty or even forty years previously. In an assessment, sixty years later, of an airman who had been involved in a heavy landing of an aircraft during WWII, it was very difficult to reconcile the history that he provided with his orthopaedic conditions that could be identified. It turned out, the presence of a visible link was irrelevant. The Department of Veterans' Affairs had already accepted liability, and the reporter's role was simply to assess his functional impairment according to the Comcare Guides.

It seemed that the lily was being gilded because there was no true causal link.

It demonstrates that when briefing an expert, it is important to be particularly precise with instructions. If a lawyer who acts for the plaintiff fears that such a nexus might be tenuous, it may be best to avoid it. Conversely, for a defendant's lawyer, this could be an excellent point at which to start investigation, despite prior acceptance of a condition, its extent or its cause.

17

LEAD ARTICLE

Horses For Courses

Despite the undesirability of revisiting issues, there are some that are so important as to justify reiteration in a different context.

When choosing an expert for an opinion required for litigation, it is imperative that the chosen one has the necessary training, experience and competence in addition to formal qualification alone. Unfortunately, the obligation rests with whomever is seeking the report to ensure this in respect of the particular case. Some experts will not tell you when they do not have the requisite capacity to provide a suitable service for the particular demand.

The most unfortunate error is committed occasionally when an Occupational Health Physician strays into the field of orthopaedic surgery other than in a superficial way. The reasons are sometimes mysterious. Lack of insight could be one. Whatever the explanation, an Occupational Health Physician is usually not equipped to comment with clarity, confidence or cogency on complex orthopaedic maladies. Their incompetence is apparent at many levels.

Like the rest of us, Occupational Physicians have limitations. The details provided in the history that they recount are frequently inadequate to assist in an orthopaedic diagnosis. Their clinical examination is often equally lacking depth and accuracy. Their diagnosis is often borrowed from another source or report. When its validity depends on the quality of the source, it should be acknowledged. Their final analysis, including impairment assessment, is sometimes grossly inaccurate.

Registered Orthopaedic Surgeons trained in this country or who have obtained the Fellowship of the Royal Australasian College of Surgeons and are members of the Australian Orthopaedic Association, have climbed a very high mountain to achieve that status. Their study, experience, registrarships and examination processes are stringent, tortuous and very thorough. Such a Fellowship holder possesses very high skills in the understanding and treatment of orthopaedic pathologies. These lauding adjectives apply equally to Orthopaedic Surgeons trained and practising in many other countries.

Practitioners without this Fellowship are less skilled, less reliable and less able in this field. The same principle applies to any other specialty. It is particularly unwise to use a specialist in a peripheral discipline to comment on matters that are principally of an orthopaedic nature. Of course, this does not detract from that expert to rely on the effect of orthopaedic conditions on matters within that person's own specialist field. The caveat is that full reference and identification is made to the sources and content of the orthopaedic facts that are assumed and relied on from such sources in the formulation of that advice. If the correctness of the sources is discountenanced, the validity of the advice based on it may be affected. The essential point in this context is that such a person relying on controversial orthopaedic issues as a basis for other advice should not pretend to be able to assess the orthopaedic issues personally.

That is not to say that there is no important place for Occupational Health Physicians, who have considerable experience in industrial medicine, workplace health and safety issues, epidemiological analyses and contributions to employment welfare. That is their sphere, where, to the same extent, orthopaedic specialists should fear to tread. This principle applies to all specialties.

Well-produced reports by experts in their field will usually have congruous essential threads. There will be little variation, little room for manoeuvre and little argument that cannot be resolved in a conclave or in mediation. Then, any need to progress to trial should be rare, costs contained and the anguish of plaintiffs diminished. This smooth professional course towards a solution may be disrupted by a poorly informed orthopaedic opinion of an Occupational Health Physician.

CASE VIGNETTE

Farm Accidents

Agricultural accidents are becoming more common and more serious. I was a victim. I fell while riding a Segway X2 on a farm track. I sustained a distressing gravel rash on his forehead and his chest struck the handlebars on the ground, causing a haemopneumothorax. In controlled factory environments or large construction sites in the city, safety regulations and practices designed to mitigate risk are strictly required. That is not the case on the average farm. Undue interference in agricultural activities is undesirable, but this is one area where greater regulation would probably help to save lives, reduce the frequency and severity of injuries and help preserve the funding corpus required for national health care.

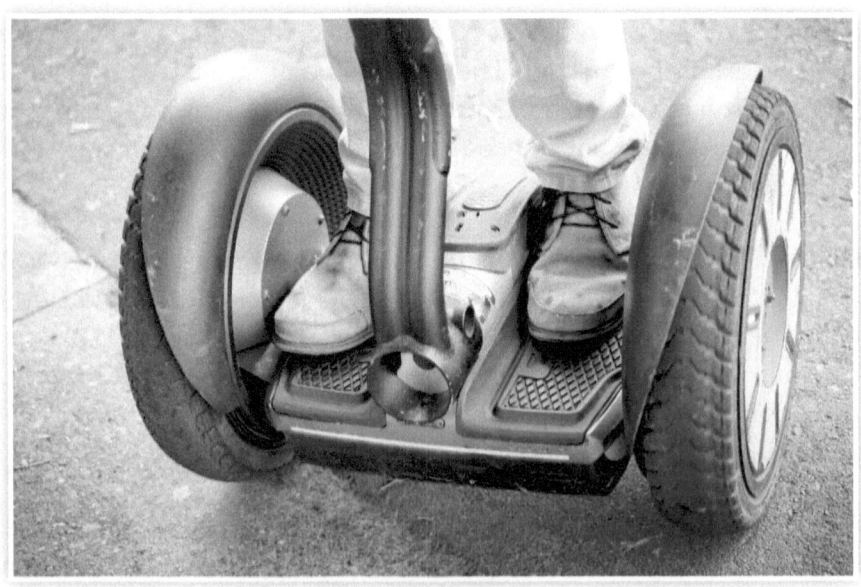

GENERAL ADVICE

Medical Negligence - The Most Bitter Pill Of All

In the medicolegal sphere forty years ago, less than 10% of a practice dealt specifically with issues of medical negligence. That ratio was predicated by the relatively low frequency of medical misadventure, the relatively high incidence of workplace and road traffic accidents, and a certain disinclination of patients to sue their doctor. But, as the younger generation becomes more populous and vocal, and the incidence of lawyers' contingency fees proliferates, the old-fashioned respect for medical practitioners will diminish. Medical negligence issues will arise more frequently. My practice in providing medical reports is now totally related to medical negligence and is engaged virtually equally by plaintiffs and defendants.

Medical school training has changed dramatically over the last few years. The National Orthopaedic Training Programme has the virtues of breadth, depth and intricacy. The expectations placed upon trainees prior to their consultancy is quite inspiring. Many are already exhibiting talents that exceed those of some of the earlier generation. With their greater knowledge and experience comes the potential for reducing medical negligence. It will not be a directly proportional equation, but the link is probably stronger than merely a grandiose wish.

In investigating and expressing an opinion on a medical negligence claim, it is important to separate expected complications from perceptions of a practitioner's under-performance. On the other hand, there are occasions when a surgeon might select the correct operation and perform it appropriately with due skill and care in the peri-operative period, but have a dramatic failure by post-operative omission to follow up astutely and carefully.

A Salutary Lesson

A patient had undergone shoulder surgery, which outwardly appeared to be very well done. Unfortunately, surveillance of her post-operative condition until her next follow up visit, six weeks later, had been delegated by her treating Orthopaedic Surgeon to a General Practitioner who was ill-equipped and under-skilled for such a task. By the time she re-presented to her Orthopaedic Surgeon, her shoulder joint was badly infected and full of pus. Had she been seen sooner, investigated appropriately. and managed aggressively, her outcome would have been much better. The case is pending in the Court. I fully expect her to be successful with her claim.

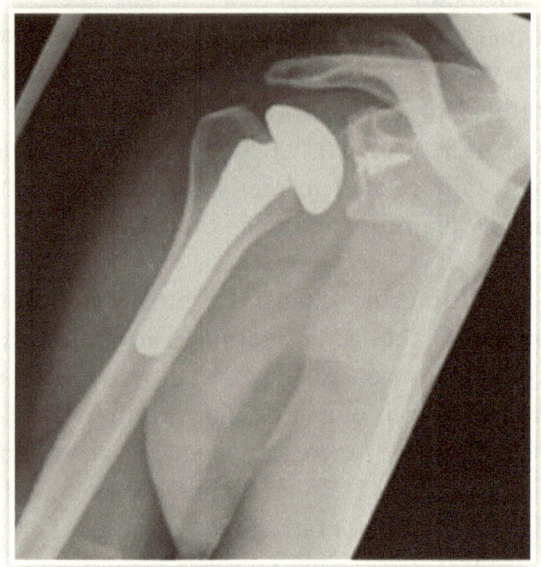

A right total shoulder replacement

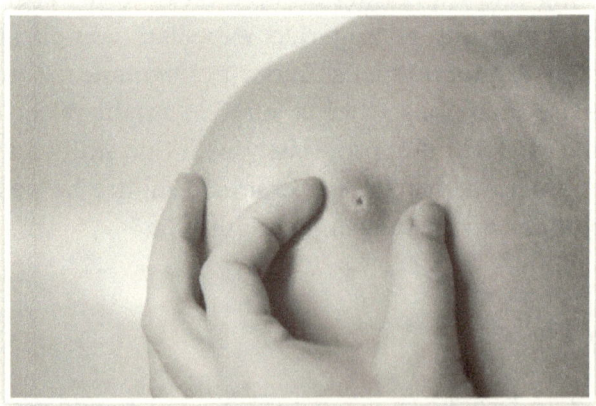

Pus draining from a sinus

LEAD ARTICLE

What Does The Future Hold?

Over the last three or four decades, the medical response to tortious personal injury and medical negligence claims has been evolving slowly but inexorably. Whereas the liaison between the medical and legal professions on such matters was once rather loose and relatively unpredictable, the entire relationship has become tighter, better controlled, and more certain.

Years ago, an elderly and highly respected practitioner in the field decried the use of any form of reference text or scale and relied simply on "a feeling", an informed intuition, as to what an impairment was likely to be. That was the percentage that he expressed. He was occasionally challenged in cross-examination, and sometimes by the Bench, but he relied upon his presence, his persona, his reputation, and his charisma to carry the day. Things have changed. I would not expect to get away with that today! Transparency and predictability for all are to be lauded.

The last decade or so has found the process more efficient with the enactment of the Civil Liability Act and the Personal Injury Proceedings Act (or their equivalents) in various jurisdictions. By introducing the 'greater than 5% permanent impairment' rule, workers insurance authorities have also been of some assistance in excluding those claims that are probably unmeritorious.

There has also been much greater specialisation by legal firms in the personal injury field and though there are still some firms that deal with either side of a claim, exclusivity is now much more common so that a firm will take only plaintiff or defendant work. This has considerably contributed to efficiency.

These beneficial evolutionary changes should continue far. On the legal side, legislative changes will be required for personal injuries sustained in driverless car collisions. With the advent of artificial intelligence, serious issues could appear, such as who is liable if its use leads to injuries? To what does the duty of care apply? Workplace health and safety regulations are stringent, arguably too much so.

On the medical side, the almost ubiquitous presence of closed-circuit television surveillance cameras has laid bare false claims of injury mechanisms. Further, if immigration enlarges, as has happened in Germany, our workplaces could contain a greater proportion of unskilled and, in that way and to that extent, theoretically unprotected workers.

Regardless of the direction in which the pendulum swings, there will be a need for experts in professional matters. Advocates and medicolegal experts are likely to remain in demand.

CASE VIGNETTE

Assessing Spinal Injuries Using The AMA 5 Guides

Chapter 15 of the AMA 5 Guides explains specifically that whenever possible, the Diagnosis Related Estimate (DRE) method should be employed. For example, if there is a fracture of L3 that has given rise to a loss of 30% of normal anterior body height, the assessor would refer to Table 15-3 on page 384. Fractures that give rise to a loss of 25%-50% of normal anterior body height qualify for DRE Lumbar Category

3 with a range of 10%-13% of whole person function. That range allows the assessor to make some allowance for associated continuing pain and discomfort. A patient who has sustained such a fracture but is otherwise relatively unscathed, would be assessed at the lower limit of the range and given a 10% whole person impairment rating. Conversely, another patient with that same fracture but who has nearly constant pain and considerable difficulties with a broad spectrum of activities of daily living, may rate at the upper limit of that range and qualify for a 13% impairment assessment.

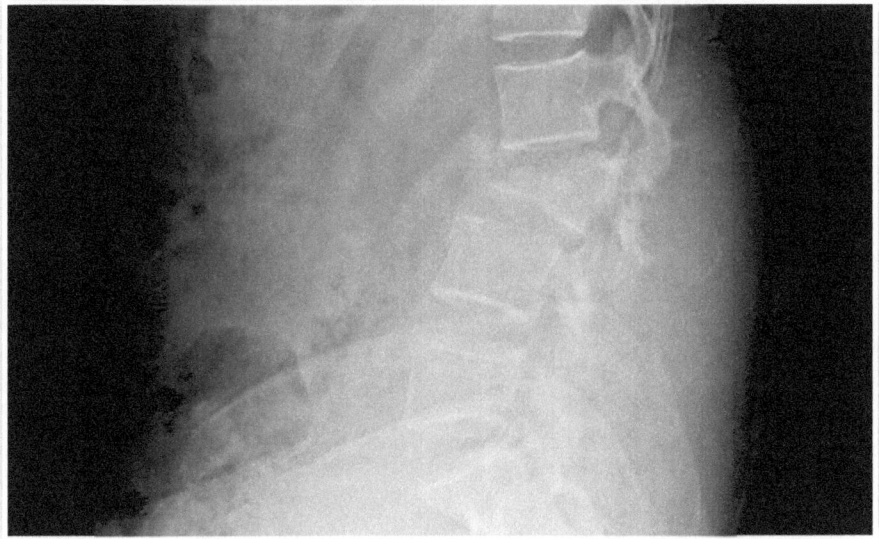

Severe anterior compression fracture involving L3

Diagnosis Related Estimates vs Range Of Motion Method

If because of the same accident a patient has more than one fracture within the lumbar spine, with, say, a loss of 30% of anterior body height at L2 because of a compression fracture, and a further loss of 10% of anterior body height at L3, the AMA 5 Guides would instruct the assessor to use the "Range of Motion" (ROM) method. This is best outlined in Table 15-7. It appears on page 404. The fracture at L2 (a loss of 30% of anterior body height) would qualify for a loss of 7% of whole person function. The fracture at L3 with a loss of 10% of anterior body height would qualify for a loss of 5% of whole person function. Together, they yield a loss of 12% of whole person function. In addition, allowances must be made for any restrictions in range of motion. Tables 15-8 and 15-9 make those allowances for losses of flexion, extension and lateral flexion to the right or left. This is a more complex analysis, but it is mandated by the AMA 5 Guides because there is more than one affected segment within that same region of the injured spine.

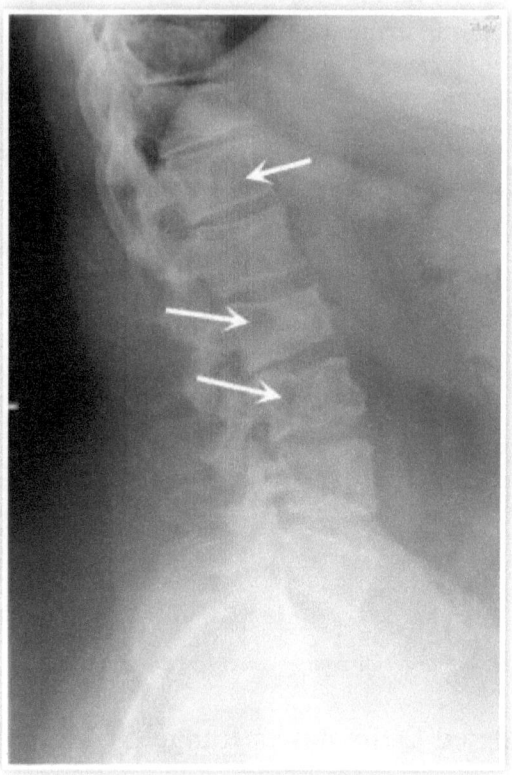

The bottom two arrows indicate the L2 and L3 fractured segments

Remember though, if there was a fracture in the cervical spine, a fracture in the thoracic spine and a fracture in the lumbar spine (3 fractures in total but all in different regions) the assessor would still use the Diagnosis Related Estimate Category (DRE) method and refer to Tables 15-5, 15-4 and 15-3 respectively. It is only when there is more than one segmental level in the same region (cervical, thoracic or lumbar) that Table 15-7 (ROM method) is used.

GENERAL ADVICE

Tips For Conversations, Whether Spoken or Written

The dramatic difference in modes of delivery between legal practitioners and medical practitioners is striking.

With some exceptions, in the presentation of their evidence, legal practitioners may stride to the podium, extract a thick folder of typed pages and begin reading from or using it as a prompt, with some occasional variation or inflection. A supercilious eyebrow may even be used for emphasis. In general terms though, it is head down and full steam ahead from start to finish. It is a valid method in the process of, not only presentation, but also of persuasion, which is a duty of an advocate.

The role, and consequent obligation, and therefore, suitable methodology of presentation of medical practitioners as witnesses are quite different. They will often have an aide-memoire, such as notes taken contemporaneously with or soon after their examinations, and some means of further explaining what they are expressing, such as a PowerPoint presentation. Then, each slide should beneficially bear a few key words in bold print or a diagram for ease in its identification in order to have a smooth process. The text of the evidence should be succinct. Medical practitioner witnesses are usually free to speak "off the cuff" in direct response to questions on specific points, and occasionally referring obliquely to their aides-memoire or the screen. Anatomical models are also sometimes used. The evidence consists of their opinions rather than the questions posed so that the responses are more engaging and educational. While the responses are facilitated by the direction provided by the questions and have no more purpose of answering to the point, the questions, on the other hand, must be formulated in a testing way, and with an ultimate persuasive strategic purpose behind them.

The same general reasoning applies to the form of written reports. They should be clearly and strictly informative, without any element of persuasion. Headings, subheadings and numbered paragraphs are useful to exemplify and clarify important points.

A few reporting experts produce simply about a half dozen typed pages, single spaced in small type and with few or no headings. The opinions can be difficult to discern. Instead, it is a pleasure to read a report that is laid out clearly, objectively and fairly progresses sequentially through the case, and concludes with a justified and well-explained opinion. Whether I agree or not becomes irrelevant. All the pleasure is in the reading.

LEAD ARTICLE

Trick or Treat?

The expression, "claim farming", relates to some law firms' hunting for work in potential personal injury claims. The "no win, no fee" proliferation is an example. As another sign, I received a cold telephone call from a lawyer following my lodging a claim for minor vehicle damage. After I indicated that no personal injury had been sustained, the caller terminated the call abruptly. It was redolent of the days of "ambulance chasers".

A national hardware retailer gave a staff directive against permitting the sale of open sausage sandwiches at their outlets. "Sausage sizzles" are typically operated at such venues by small, "not-for-profit" community groups to raise funds for worthwhile service endeavours. The retailer reasonably perceived undeserved risks of claims for personal injury which could adversely affect normal operations. The hardware retailer was subjected to irrational criticism, despite seemingly having a genuine concern for the disturbance of involvement of a possibly unmeritorious lawsuit in a growingly litigious society.

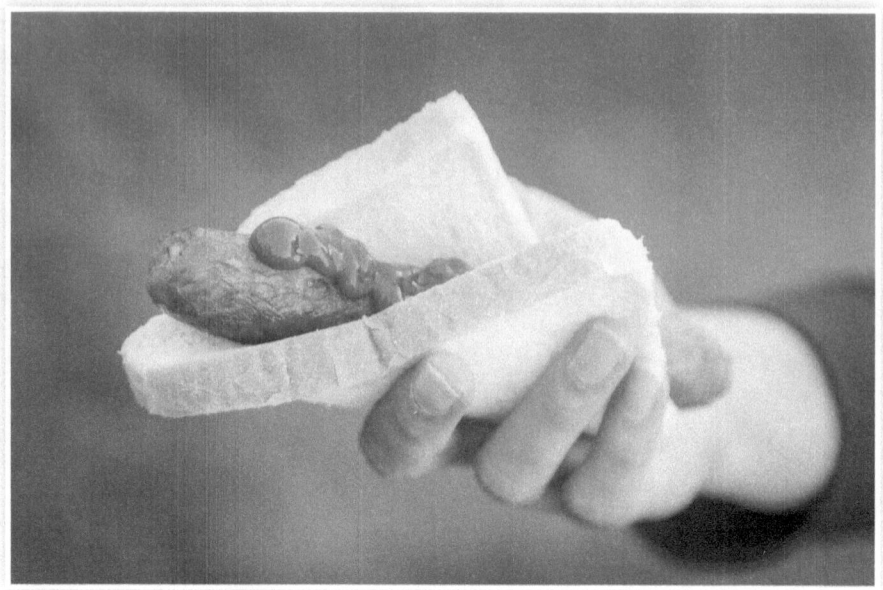

While genuine cases exist and should be suitably compensated, the danger to be avoided is the threat posed by the contrivance of false claims for incompensable injuries, which are then exaggerated as part of the dishonest scheme. Shoppers' slipping on lettuce leaves, grapes and spilt liquid in supermarkets are classical instances of possibly dubious claims. The worse feature of this is the ease with which the occasion of the injury may be concocted, but at least the medical discrepancies may be better identified

What Does This Mean?

The figures are rather alarming. Unmeritorious compensation claims contributed to an increase of AUD$75 per year in the cost of Compulsory Third Party insurance coverage for every vehicle in western countries.

Vexatious personal injury claims encouraged by "claim farming" are already affecting the insurance industry and consequently, of necessity, premiums that must be paid for the protection provided by insurance cover.

The legal and medical professions may have an increase in business because of this growth of litigation in this field, but it would be a spurious benefit overall. We all should remember that the path to success in medicolegal litigation can sometimes be fraught with serious dangers.

CASE VIGNETTE

Pre-existent Abnormalities Can Be Made Worse

A 25-year-old male cyclist was dislodged and landed awkwardly, sustaining a dislocation of his right patella (the kneecap moves to the outside of the lower end of the thigh bone). This is usually a particularly painful injury. Sometimes it reduces spontaneously at the scene, but more commonly it requires transfer to a hospital for a closed reduction under a neurolept anaesthetic. He required that closed reduction.

The joint had not been normal prior to this accident. He had suffered from generalised ligamentous laxity or, as it is sometimes called, "double- jointedness". In this condition, ligaments that stabilise joints are relatively long or lax, so that the range of motion in almost every joint in the body is more than normal. It predisposes the person to joint instabilities, subluxations (partial dislocations) or even frank dislocations. In addition, his natural kneecap was riding higher than normal, and well outside the restraining groove on the lower end of his thigh bone. The kneecap was also smaller than normal and the same groove on the femur was shallower than normal. He was also knock-kneed. In essence therefore, he had several features of predisposition to dislocation, but despite these quite powerful factors, he had never suffered any adverse symptoms. The accident caused the joint to be troublesome, and without it, he may never have suffered a dislocation.

Because of the uncertainty of the future arising from his predisposition to injury, quantifying his impairment and disability arising from the accident was theoretically complicated, but should not have been. Regardless or otherwise of those factors, he was subjected to a single specific traumatic event and suffered an identifiable compensable injury. This is exactly what the Court ultimately found. Any allowance in respect of future losses arising from future circumstances that included his predisposition as a factor, so that the future losses caused by the subject accident would no longer be incurred or would be diminished would be a matter for the Court. The only medicolegal factor would be the degree of predisposition, associated with its likelihood for natural progression in a way that might interfere with the assessment of loss attributable to the subject accident.

GENERAL ADVICE

Does A Contralateral Joint Suffer By Favouring An Injured Joint?

Patients who have an injured hip, knee, elbow, or shoulder sometimes subsequently complain of an "injury" involving the contralateral joint (the same joint on the other side of the body) by virtue of any favouring of the injured joint.

Orthopaedic literature is quite firm. Such secondary injuries are almost universally fanciful. In the absence of any additional or specific injury, there is no relationship.

Even if a patient is imposing greater stress on an uninjured and pristine limb, it is capable of bearing any increased stress, which should be absorbed quite easily. Further, because of the state of the injured part, the patient may be less active than usual, so that the contralateral uninjured joint is probably doing less work than usual.

Dismissing this misconception early may save considerable time, trouble and expense.

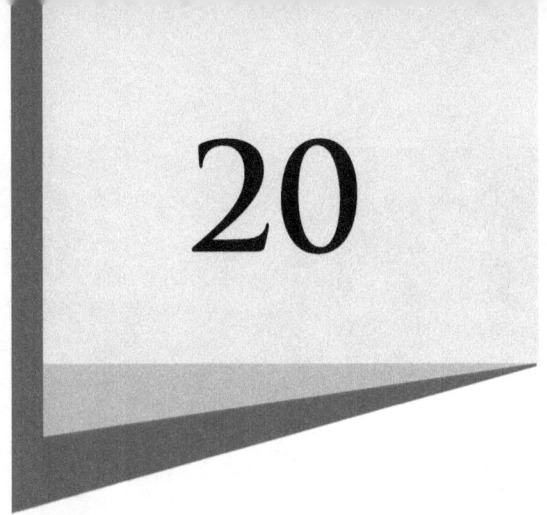

LEAD ARTICLE

Same Word But Different Connotations

The words "fracture" or "break", when applied to a bone, are basically synonymous.

In the course of his work, a middle-aged male claimant had jumped from a height of some 900mm (about 3 ft), had landed on both feet, and did not overbalance further. He felt a twinge of pain in his back and felt a small pain in his right groin. He thought little of it. Over the next few weeks, his back pain settled but his groin pain persisted and increased. On x-ray examination, the radiographic images demonstrated long-standing, pre-existent avascular necrosis of the femoral head (the death of a wedge-shaped segment of bone in the ball on the upper end of his thigh bone). That process had been present and progressive for many months, if not years before this episode. The cause of the avascularity (or loss of blood supply) is often never determined. Importantly, it was not due to his work practices in general, nor this minor jump.

In addition, there was a small fracture identified within this avascular or dead zone within the femoral head. The pain did not resolve but rather increased. That fracture was incapable of healing. The claimant had a total hip replacement costing around AUD$50,000.

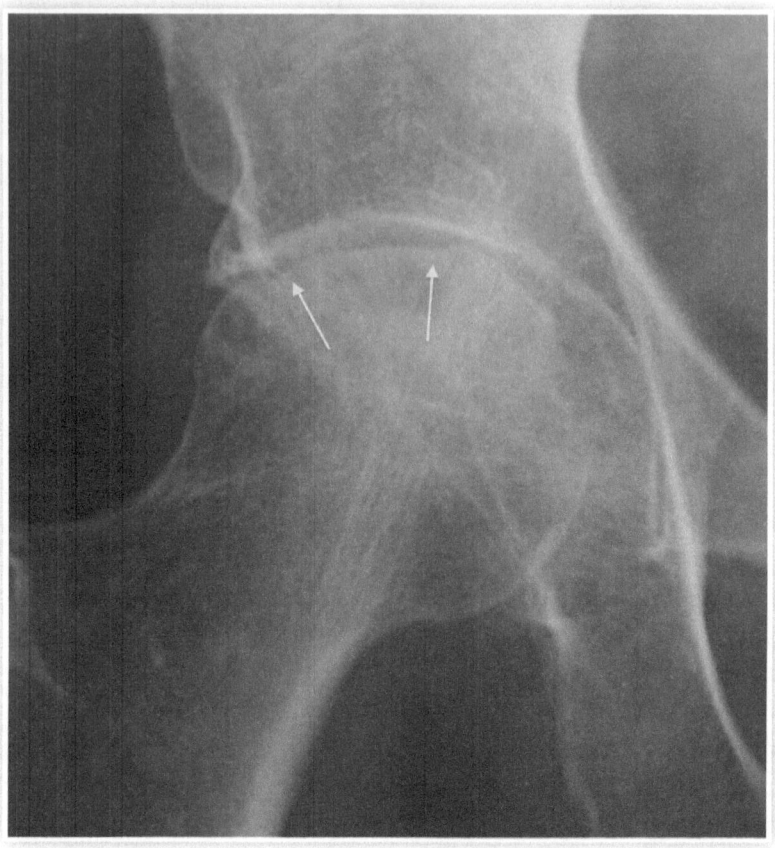

The arrows show the margins of the depressed fracture in the avascular segment

He lodged a claim, and his solicitor accepted his categoric denial of prior discomfort in his hip or the right groin, believing that although the hip might not have exhibited completely normal radiographic features, the sudden change in his client's condition must have been linked in some way to the event. He contended, on behalf of the claimant, that the "fracture" was new, and caused by the jump.

On the other side, the defendant's solicitor fixed upon the word, "fracture". He knew that fractures could occur from massive or severe insults, and assumed that all fractures were caused by excessive loads or serious trauma. He further assumed this fracture showing on the x-ray of the hip of a man who had jumped such a short distance was not due to the relevant "accident".

The Mechanics Involved

Normal bone is a living organ, quite resilient and elastic. It can absorb stresses, strains and excessive loads, including a jump from a height of 3 ft, with ease. In contrast, dead bone lacks that resilience, and is therefore unable to withstand normal stresses and strains adequately and as competently. Over time (weeks, months or even years), the devitalised bone will tend to collapse and fracture. This is a "pathological fracture" where the structural failure occurs in abnormal (weaker) bone through the application of perfectly normal stresses. Furthermore, this isolated "trivial" event may also have precipitated the "pathological fracture" at a time sooner than reasonably expected.

So What?

He was 49 years old and much younger than the usual patient who undergoes a hip replacement. Most hip replacements perform extremely well statistically and he could expect a failure rate of about 0.5% per annum for the first 20 years. He had only a 10% chance of requiring a revision procedure before he was 69 years old, thereafter, the revision rate climbs more rapidly. As he had a life expectancy of 30 years following his joint surgery, he had grounds for concern.

Quantum

The Court accepted that his employer was at least partly responsible for the outcome. Neither the claimant nor his employer was aware of the pre-existing avascular changes in his femoral head. Nor did either of them consider that such a trivial event would have such a dramatic effect. Regardless of the sequence, causation was accepted. But, as for the correct description of the mechanics of his injury, insofar as it was relevant to his loss, and his award of damages, in this context, a "fracture" is not necessarily "a fracture". The word, "fracture", is the same, but their connotations are very different.

The claimant's surgical intervention had been hastened by some years, he had been exposed to a greater likelihood of requiring further surgery, and he was at additional risk of potential complications. Financial losses were suffered also because of his reduced working capacity and uncertainty of employment.

CASE VIGNETTE

Whom Would You Get To Do Your Hip Replacement?

Lawyers typically know which fellow practitioners are competent and those who are not. Medical practitioners should be the same, but they are not. The difference is probably due to the public exposure of a lawyer's work, at least, to an opposing lawyer, but more often because of public performance. They say, "Doctors bury their mistakes". That's a very unkind view but it can be difficult to relate outcome with medical competence. This is especially true with surgeons. Many doctors will require the assistance of surgical intervention from time to time. The real question then is, whom to trust?

This harbours more difficulty than might be apparent. A preference for a certain hospital or a specific medical device will narrow the choice. Personality may have a role, but ultimately, the best selection is an expert technician with a low complication rate and a reputation for results that yield an excellent long-term outcome.

Not many other doctors witness surgeons in the act of operating. General practitioners, the referral source, rarely see surgeons in action. Surgical trainees are better positioned, since they assist many consultants in a variety of settings. Consultants themselves are often busy at their own activities, and do not spend much time in the presence of their colleagues in the operating theatre.

Is There A Reliable Reference Source?

The Australian Orthopaedic Association National Joint Replacement Registry (AOANJRR) collates outcome data following hip replacements, knee replacements, shoulder replacements and knee joint anterior cruciate ligament reconstructions on an annual basis. Other countries, such as Sweden, Denmark, Canada, the USA and the United Kingdom, also have registries. The rates of contribution of data by Australian surgeons are close to 100%. Because longitudinal analyses are possible, by asking a surgeon how she or he fares at a national level, an observer can determine which surgeons are performing better than the national average. It should aid the choice considerably.

Despite a best choice, not all outcomes are successful. Complications can and do occur, and some surgeons commit technical errors. Inadvertent lengthening of the limb, significantly altering joint mechanics, and damaging sensory nerves are three.

GENERAL ADVICE

Staying Calm Under Fire

Most medical practitioners are comfortable within their clinical environment, but that equilibrium does not necessarily extend to the court room. Giving evidence-in-chief is usually straightforward. Cross-examination, however, can be more stressful.

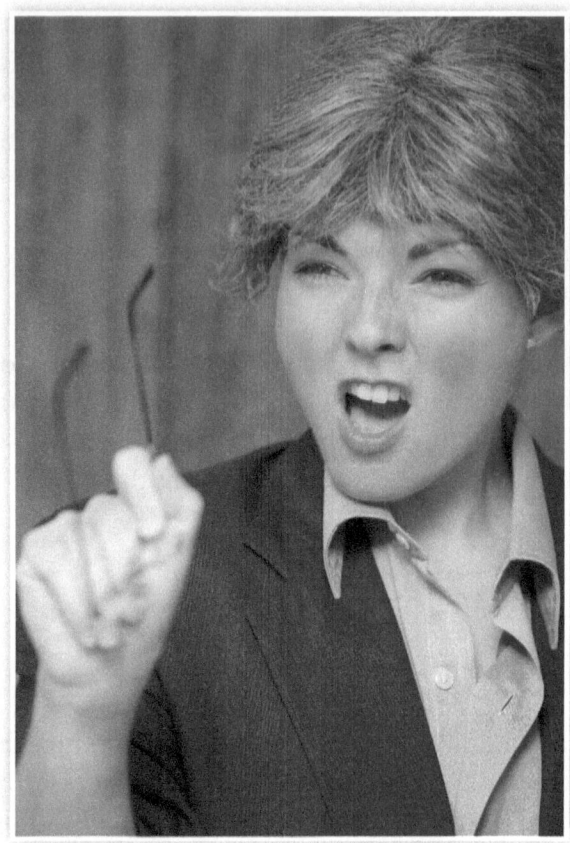

Some barristers can be very testy

It is sometimes wise for a lawyer to provide some pre-court advice to a medical expert who is to give evidence. Explaining the desirability of considering opposite opinions, forewarning of likely contentious issues, and a brief description of relevant personality traits of the judge and opposing counsel are useful.

It is the sole task of an expert witness to assist the Court, and not to take the side of either of the parties. Although Counsel will conduct the questioning, the expert's responses are provided for the Bench, which also appreciates commonsense.

Unfortunately, experts sometimes engage in argument, obfuscation, irritability and intransigence. All are undesirable. Skilled counsel have an ability to agitate even some of the calmest of experts. With agitation comes haste, fluster, ill-conceived answers and underperformance. Prejudices and egocentric behaviours sometimes emerge. These damage the force of that expert's evidence. An expert witness' focus should be to ensure that the court understands the opinion expressed, and why it has been formed. Acceptance of that opinion is a matter for the court, which may have evidence unknown to the expert.

There are several strategies for the desirable state of staying calm. They include pausing and reflecting appropriately before answering, speaking reasonably slowly, answering the questions directly, resisting rephrasing of questions by examining counsel, and retaining suitable humility. All help with equanimity.

LEAD ARTICLE

Clinical Examinations And Sexual Boundaries

Clinical examination is a vital part of any medical assessment. Those that require an examination of an intimate nature are uncommon. Views of what will constitute an intimate examination will vary from one observer to another, but it generally involves the clinical examination, both visual and manual, of the breasts and genitalia. It may extend to digital penetration of the vagina or rectum. There will be some occasions when a rectal examination is necessary to an orthopaedic assessment to assess anal tone. Patients who suffer with cauda equina syndrome, that is, where the lower nerve roots of the spinal cord are being compromised, can suffer with faecal, and sometimes urinary, incontinence and lack anal tone.

Neurological examinations of the lower limbs usually focus upon the nerve roots that are exiting from the spinal cord numbered L1 - L5 and S1-S2. The genitalia are supplied by the nerve roots S2 to S4 inclusive, so they rarely require examination. It is perfectly possible to assess the neurological status of a lower limb thoroughly without engaging in any intimate examination.

If, however, doubt ever exists, a chaperone, such as the practitioner's secretary, should always be present in the consulting room during the examination. Most female patients would welcome such support, and it must always be offered. If there is any concern, the presence of a chaperone should be insisted upon by the medical practitioner. There may be occasions where claimants present without even underwear, and then, clinical gowns should always be provided.

The Australian Health Practitioners Regulation Agency (AHPRA), the Australian Medical Association (AMA), and the medical defence organisations within Australia all publish guidelines and recommendations concerning intimate examinations and the presence of a chaperone or support person. Other countries have similar regulatory bodies and codes. It is the practitioner's responsibility to understand their requirements, and to ensure that they are met. Patient dignity is paramount. Inappropriate comments, sexual touching, and activities that result in embarrassment, are never acceptable.

CASE VIGNETTE

Temporal Links Are Not Always Important

A man seventy-two years of age gave a history of having fallen from a tram. The tram was at a standstill, and he was alighting on its correct side at a designated stop. He was unencumbered, walked without aids, had his hands free, and was cognitively aware of his surroundings. The gap between the floor of the tram and the platform was 225mm. Despite this constellation of reassuring features, his right knee joint gave way as he placed his right foot on the concrete platform below. He remembered twisting his torso ever so slightly in a clockwise direction, losing his balance, and falling onto his right side. He did not lose consciousness although remembers feeling extremely embarrassed. He was travelling alone and it appears that he was ignored by passers-by. He was able to gather his wits, clamber to his feet and proceed on foot for the block and a half to his hotel.

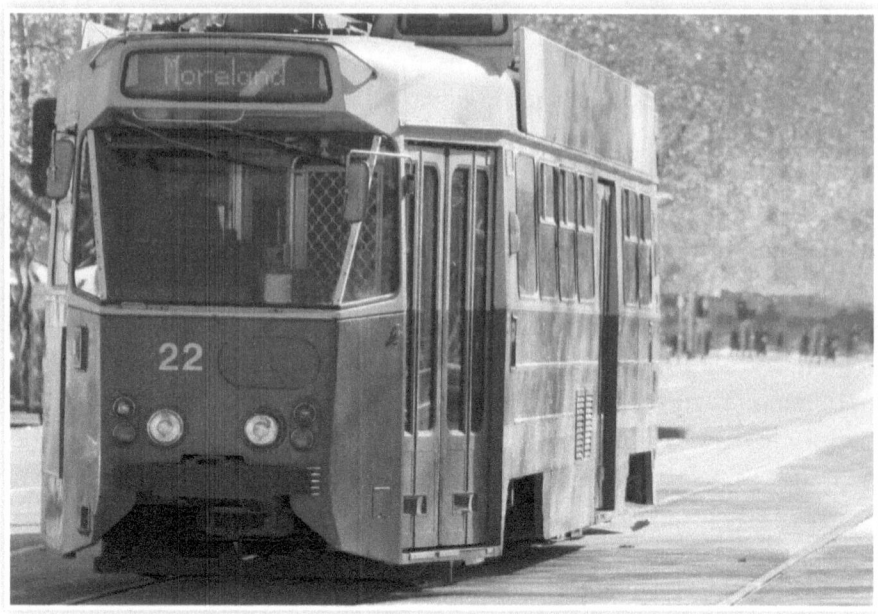

The incident occurred just after 5:00pm, allowing sufficient time for two glasses of wine before dinner. Near the end of the second glass, his embarrassment faded and he became angry. Why did it happen? Whose fault was it? What if he had been seriously injured? Apart from this emotional response, he thought little more of the incident and had no real pain in his right knee.

The following morning however, the knee joint was painful, it appeared to be mildly swollen and his anger piqued.

He returned to his home four days later. There was still a bit of a niggle in the knee, so he consulted with his local medical officer. Radiographs were performed and he was shown to be suffering with quite severe osteoarthritis in all three compartments of the joint.

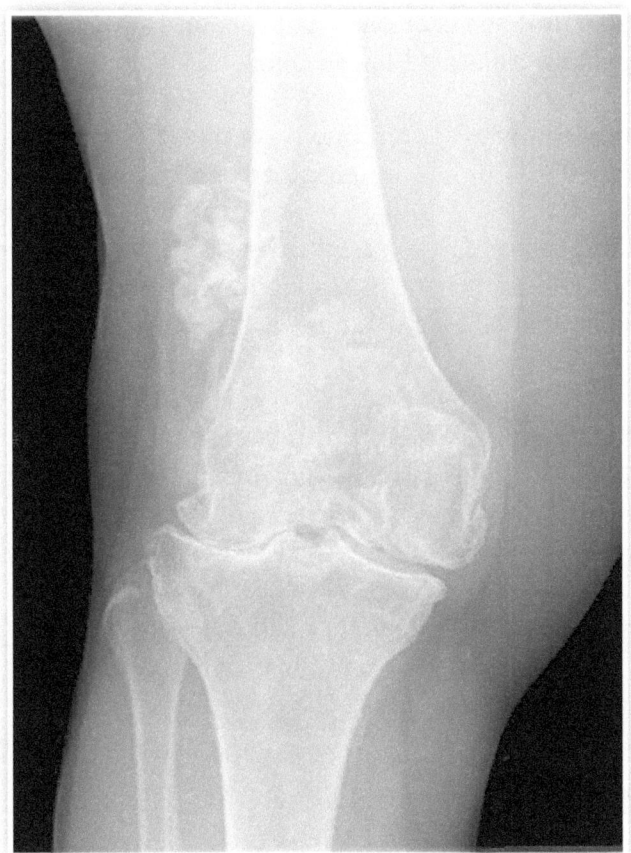
Severe arthritis involving the entire joint. Several loose bodies.

Looking down at the joint, there is a compartment on the inside, another on the outside and a third behind the knee cap. His radiographs showed that the joint spaces in all three compartments were severely narrowed, the end plates of the thigh bone and the shin bone were quite sclerotic (appearing white on the x-ray), large spurs had formed at the margins of the joints, and there were several defects in the bone, probably in the form of osteoarthritic cysts or geodes. Surprisingly, the x-rays also revealed large ossified loose bodies within the confines of the joint.

He was adamant that he was completely unaware that his knee was so severely diseased. Instead, he focused upon the temporal link between the incident that had occurred as he stumbled just a bit when alighting from the tram, and the later onset of his pain. He was convinced that the temporal link translated to causation.

He found a lawyer who agreed, and was prepared to act on a "no-win, no-fee" basis, and sent him for a medicolegal examination.

Stranger things have happened, in that serious degenerative changes showing on an x-ray had, it was claimed, hitherto been completely asymptomatic. It is still highly unlikely, and outside the experience of senior observers.

It is also highly unlikely that on this occasion, the incident played a significant role in the inexorable and inevitable demise of his knee joint. It might have caused some temporary exacerbation, causing additional pain that may have focused his attention on the knee.

It did not change its natural history, did not alter either the timing or the extent of any subsequent therapy that he may require, nor is he worthy of any compensation.

GENERAL ADVICE

Complaints To Medical Practitioner Regulatory Authorities

The process of dealing with complaints relating to medical conduct is not entirely satisfactory when they relate to opinions given by experts in medicolegal reports. Regulatory agencies are neither well equipped for, nor in possession of, a purview to comment with authority upon the opinions expressed. The resources that need to be marshalled in responding to such a complaint may be addressing matters of a medicolegal nature in a case of civil litigation and the complaint may have become a "fishing expedition", which is discouraged by the Courts. Complaints originating in bad faith may also be employed to intimidate improperly a potential witness whose evidence may be contrary to the interests of the complainant.

It is certainly the right of any person to make a complaint about such opinions but this is not the correct forum. Such complaints should be raised by the party's solicitor through a proper legal process, seeking an explanatory response, and then dealing with it appropriately according to the rules controlling litigation.

The abuse of the processes of a public utility, such as a regulatory agency, is not appropriate. This view applies equally to the legal profession. Legal service commissions are not constituted to investigate particular matters of litigation while it is in progress in a way that will provide an inappropriate benefit to a complainant who is a party to the litigation. Such agencies exist to ensure practitioners in their jurisdiction perform professionally.

22

LEAD ARTICLE

New Kids On The Block

Both France and Canada have leaders who are relatively young - "new kids on the block". They may have intellect, competence, social consciences, and political skills, but *ex hypothesi*, they are likely to lack some experience. The same can be said in medicolegal reporting. For consistent quality, age is not the prime determinant. Instead it is the time that the reporter has spent within the specialty and, within the arena. Very few experts embark upon a career in medicolegal reporting early in their medical practice. It is much more common, though not universal, that they do so near the end of their clinical careers. It is a way of feathering their superannuation nest, funding unprofitable hobbies, and keeping an otherwise ageing mind active. Because of their experience and standing, they are desirable choices by lawyers who are preparing a case involving their expertise. However, some of them lack the necessary skill set. Some tend to pontificate, some assume facts without satisfactory evidence, and others are simply insufficiently aware of the intricacies of a legal process.

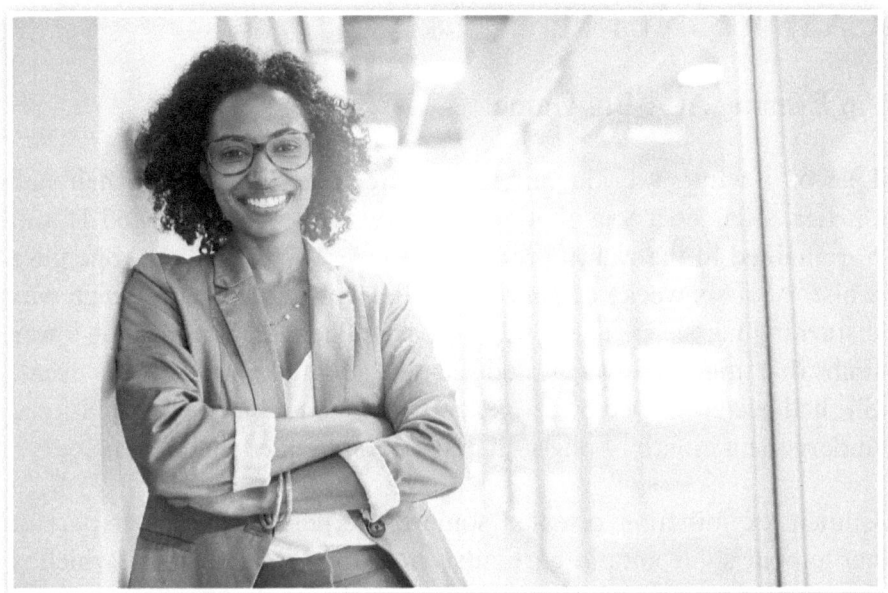

Within the alternative range, not every young newcomer will have some inadequacy, though some will be underdone. Those who pursue the career purely for its financial rewards might not necessarily be best. Their reliance for their personal reputation on a broker or a commercial report-procurement firm could predicate undesirable features of attitude.

The problem then is how does a claimant's solicitor choose the correct medical expert, at the correct time, and for the correct case?

Whom To Choose?

The answer is to inquire carefully. Former results are important. There is no formal audit of medicolegal performance in the personal injury jurisdiction, but general reputation from various sources will usually provide suitable background information.

It is sometimes worth some additional cost, waiting a little longer and being discerning to ensure that the report obtained can reasonably be relied upon.

CASE VIGNETTE

An Evening At A Big Game

Late on a winter's Friday afternoon, a couple, probably in their late thirties, attended a consultation. Their two children, boys aged 11 and 8, remained in the waiting room. The wife was the patient. She gave a history of six-weeks of almost constant lower back pain which was disturbing her sleep. There was no particular radiation into the lower limbs that might have suggested sciatica, and no known inciting event. She had been reviewed by her general practitioner on several occasions, undergone a month of physiotherapy, and attended a chiropractor.

Clinical examination revealed some tenderness in the lower part of her lumbar spine and, in particular, near the sacroiliac joint, which is made up of the sacrum (a part of the vertebral column) medially, and the hemi-pelvic wing, or ilium, laterally. Her radiographs of the lumbar spine were unremarkable. Her CT scan examination was also within normal limits. There was no sign of any disc narrowing, disc bulging, or neural compromise

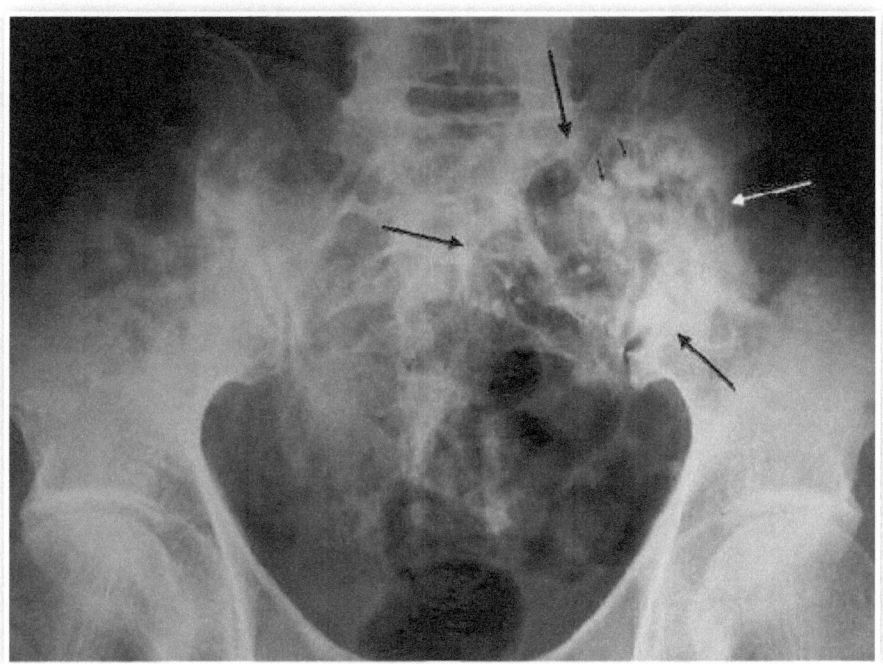

The arrows outline the destructive lesion in the sacrum

However, alarmingly, on the left side, medial to the sacroiliac joint, and involving the sacrum proper was a lesion, approximately 5cm across, and similar in appearance to a small shark bite. This was her first presentation with breast cancer, consisting of a secondary deposit in the pelvis, which was destroying bone, and heralding a premature end to her life.

Its cause and suitable treatment were clearly outside my clinical spectrum. I broke the news as gently as I could and made several telephone calls for her to be seen by both a breast surgeon and an oncologist the following morning, the Saturday. They were grateful but overwhelmed with intense grief.

As if that was not enough, the family was en route to a home match of their favourite football team, planning to dine on hamburgers on the way. Amongst their myriad distressing thoughts, this young couple was confronted with the problem of how they could break the news to their boys. An option discussed was whether to hold the news until the morrow so that the boys could enjoy the much-anticipated match. Another was to tell them, but still go to the match and try to enjoy themselves. Still another was to tell them, and simply go home.

I felt great grief for them. I'm not sure what they decided to do. It remains one of half a dozen such memories that will never fade.

GENERAL ADVICE

Educating The Experts

Issues as to how lawyers should inform their medical experts on the types of reports they need, the questions that should be answered, the issues that should be avoided and the general performance of the expert in the court atmosphere have already been discussed.

Yet another facet in which experts require education relates to periodic changes in the law and court procedures. Relevant regulations, such as those to be found in the recently enacted Personal Injuries Proceeding Act (PIPA) and the Civil Liability Act (CLA), are mostly precise and important, and adherence to them and the requirements of the Court is essential. The obligations required in a process become familiar with repeated use, but briefing-solicitors who provide written guidance in their letters of instruction should be applauded. The expert should be in no doubt on such matters.

A state Law Society Journal is a fascinating publication for a medicolegal reporter, not only for its specific attention to matters which with the reporter might need to deal, but also for its demonstration of the nature of legal thinking. The way lawyers write, think, and express themselves is intriguing. It is particularly rewarding to pay special attention to judgments of the Court of Appeal. They usually relate to matters of a commercial or criminal nature, but occasionally deal in depth with issues related to personal injuries or medical negligence. This is educational, and sometimes surprising. Some convoluted sentences are long and complex, but with inbuilt logic. The judgements referred to in footnotes are not of great interest to a medical reader, but some judgements of the High Court of Australia are of considerable relevance to medicolegal reporting. A most significant such judgment is that in *Rogers ats Whittaker*, where the plaintiff succeeded by a majority of 4 to 3!

There have been some very interesting judgements dealing with the failure of a general practitioner to call back a patient after an abnormal pap smear result, despite her being given a follow-up appointment. Another doctor was castigated for failing to offer a patient a chance to attend a surgeon with greater experience in the removal of parathyroid glands. The explanation of the general duty of care owed to a patient who may be recalcitrant in following advice is also illuminating.

Whereas medical practitioners are often invited to legal conferences as guest speakers, the converse does not happen nearly often enough. Perhaps it is time for Law Societies and Bar Associations to approach their colleges in medicine to offer their services and rain on the medical parades!

LEAD ARTICLE

Talking To Patients Or Clients

Lawyers and doctors have this duty in common. They need to converse at the commencement of the service, while establishing some form of liaison, during the process and at the end. This could be at the conclusion of the claim, or at the end of a therapeutic regimen. Some do it better than others. Most have an intelligence quotient (IQ) above average, but unfortunately, an IQ level is not necessarily associated closely with social competence. EQ, the emotional ability to engage and liaise with people, is also sometimes lacking.

Doctors routinely begin by taking a history, performing a relevantly full examination, often reviewing some ancillary investigations, and, bringing all the data elicited, hopefully make a correct diagnosis. Then, a proper therapeutic regimen can be devised and actioned. In the Law, the steps may be slightly different, and obviously have different names, but the process is probably similar in nature.

In these activities, boundaries and some barriers must be established. The barriers can be of a social, professional or sexual nature. At a social level, it is probably best not to engage too closely with a client or patient, though in verbal discourse, some characteristics of communication, such as warmth, empathy, genuineness and care, can be of use. At a professional level, aloofness is not ideal, but a retention of some polite distance can aid objectivity and make delivery of unsavoury or unhappy news easier. The need for sexual boundaries speaks for itself.

Some practitioners, especially young males in orthopaedic surgery, see expressions of warmth, empathy, genuineness and care as a sign of weakness, perhaps out of fear that such empathetic signs may be misinterpreted. It may also be feared that when complications inevitably, albeit, rarely, occur, one's ability to deal with them professionally and objectively could be compromised in some way by what has passed. With age and experience may come a belief that all such qualities are very important and should regularly and from the beginning form part of the professional discourse. In addition, a friendly exchange and interchange with patients may afford a practitioner considerable pleasure.

CASE VIGNETTE

Causation - Direct And Indirect

In a case of a male patient who had sustained an exceedingly severe compound fracture-dislocation of his ankle when his foot was almost ripped off, photographs depicted that the lower end of his talus (the ankle bone), was protruding through a large wound in his skin. His foot was dangling precariously in mid-air. Despite the passage of two or three years, five expertly performed operations, and extensive physiotherapy and rehabilitation, he remained grossly impaired and disabled. There is a question as to whether he should have had a primary below knee amputation at the time, but that was not in issue.

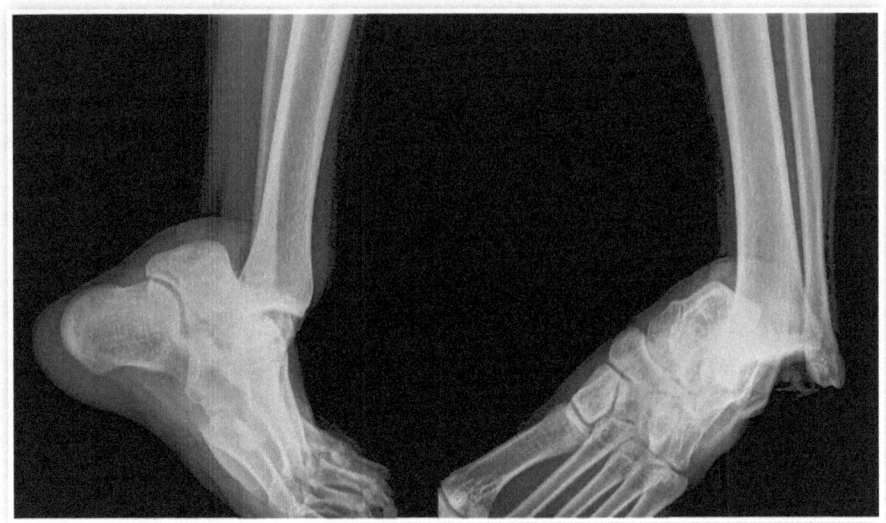

Compound fracture-dislocation of the ankle

He had begun to suffer from discomfort in the contralateral uninjured foot, and developed metatarsalgia, a condition characterised by loss of height in the distal transverse arch of the forefoot. As the metatarsal heads drop, they become closer to the plantar surface and generate pressure in the plantar pad adjacent to the shoe sole or the floor. Patients complain of a sensation of "walking on pebbles". There can be myriad causes for it.

It is tempting in this case to say that because he could not walk on his injured leg for a prolonged period, he was placing additional stresses and strains on the contralateral foot, giving rise to this indirect causation of the metatarsalgia. Temptation is insufficient, and there is no orthopaedic evidence of such a connection. In general terms, favouring one limb does not give rise to significant orthopaedic pathology in another limb. However, many plaintiffs and their lawyers hold a belief in a connection, and express disappointment when the concept is dismissed by their expert.

GENERAL ADVICE

The Opioid Epidemic

The last decade has seen a dramatic increase in the use of natural and synthetic opioids. Strong mind-altering drugs are usually prescribed as powerful analgesics. The logical implication is that they should be prescribed only for patients with severe pain. Minor analgesics should be used for pain below that threshold. The distinction is often poorly defined, but that is no excuse for lack of proper assessment and common sense. Opioids are highly addictive, which is a powerful reason to limit their use to sparingly. Unfortunately, this is not happening.

How Bad Is The Problem?

Recent publications have reported some alarming statistics in the United States of America. Of the world's population, it has approximately 5%, which, unfortunately, uses 85% of the world supply of opioids. Not only adults are addicted. Paediatric dependence is becoming increasingly common, with serious long-term ramifications. This surge is propelled by socio-economic factors, combined with genetic predispositions. Little can be done in respect of genetics, but it is possible to apply much closer scrutiny in those societies in which these medications are being distributed excessively.

In the lower socio-economic stratum in Australia, general medical practitioners are much more likely to bulk bill. That bulk billing rebate provided by the Commonwealth Medical Benefits Scheme and the Australian Government is barely sufficient to cover the costs generated in a general practice. Unsurprisingly, general practitioners who bulk bill are more likely to have shorter consultation times. As the time spent with a patient diminishes, so does any opportunity for counselling and educational dialogue. Rather than addressing issues such as depression and anxiety, and reducing the effects of chronic pain through counselling, it is easier for a general practitioner in that situation simply to acquiesce and repeat a prescription for an opioid.

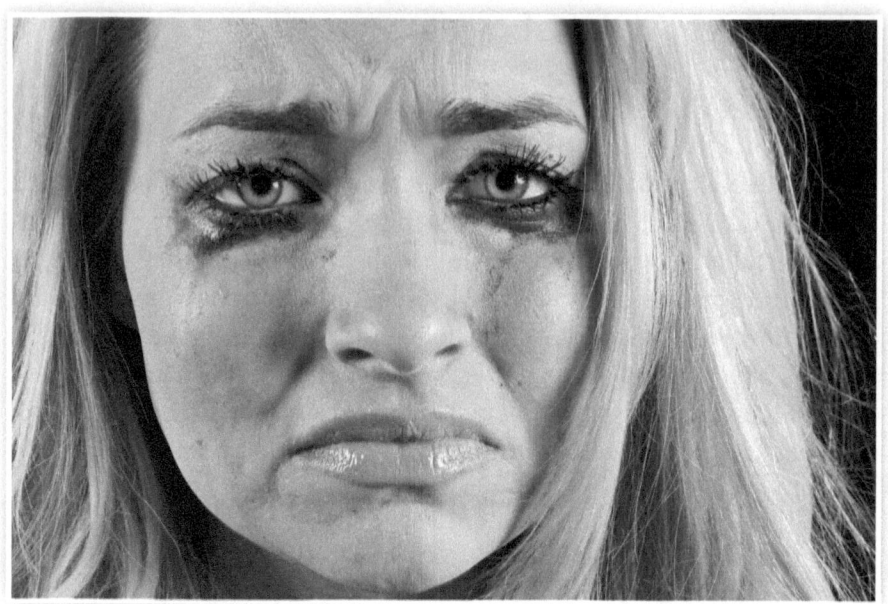

This trend is dangerous, and manifested daily through dependency, family disharmony, crime and corruption. It could be argued that the opioid epidemic is the most pressing problem facing medicine in the next decade. Personal injury litigation lawyers should not be divorced from all responsibility. They may be in a position to warn their clients, counsel relatives, and even influence the therapeutic course of their clients' medical treatment for their injuries.

LEAD ARTICLE

Most Experts Are Not Expert In Everything

This is a relatively common theme, which has already been canvassed tangentially. It is generally accepted that specialists should confine themselves to their own specialties. There are even some specialties that have focused sub-specialties that may give rise to further sensible exclusions. In orthopaedics, for example, there are specialists who respectively deal with the hand, the spine, or the foot and ankle only. Most can give a cogent general opinion on these various anatomical regions and their maladies, but there will be times when a sub-specialty opinion should be sought. This is most apparent when future therapeutic requirements are canvassed. Whilst a general orthopaedic surgeon can understand and explain the concepts of an orthopaedic condition that follows an injury, he or she may not be so confident about the latest trends in therapeutic regimens.

This problem is even more plain if, for example, a specialist, say in neurosurgery, was to comment upon shoulders or knees. Occupational Physicians also venture too far into orthopaedic waters and give misdirected advice. A cardiologist may have spent an orthopaedic term or two as a medical student or a junior house officer, but it is highly unlikely that commentary from that source on a spinal condition would be of any use to the Court. So, too, orthopaedists should properly recognize the limits of their authority to give opinions on matters beyond their specialty.

How Wide Is The Divide?

That then leads to the divide between orthopaedic surgery and psychiatry. Very few, if any, orthopaedic surgeons would be competent to provide an authoritative opinion on psychoses. Neuroses, however, may be a different matter. Surprising as it might seem, they are also human beings, and sometimes, intelligent. They understand that injured plaintiffs may have suffered physical and emotional loss, are sometimes financially compromised, and may have suffered some loss of consortium. Any of these, or a combination of some, may well and understandably cause frustration, anger, resentment, embellishment and overreaction. It is therefore tempting for the orthopaedic surgeon to stray into this field by attempting to explain a set of clinical symptoms that do not normally fit with an orthopaedically recognisable pattern by reference to such a factor. This is undesirable, and it opens the reporter who does so to valid criticism for straying into expertise which are not possessed. Such a reporter will have acted appropriately by referring to the absence of any orthopaedic association with the person's relevant complaints, and to leave it to an expert in the appropriate field to comment on psychological factors. By this means, any weakening of the force of the orthopaedic opinion given will be avoided.

CASE VIGNETTE

More Than One Way To Skin A Cat

A long spiral fracture of the femur (thigh bone) can been operatively treated with the insertion of a metal rod through the centre of the bone, with interlocking screws positioned above and below the fracture. It can sometimes be accomplished without opening the fracture site. The rod is inserted from above (or below) and alignment jigs with x-ray guidance assist in screw positioning. The rod provides longitudinal stability for the fracture and prevents angulation at the fracture site. The interlocking screws above and below provide rotary stability, and prevent the fracture from distracting.

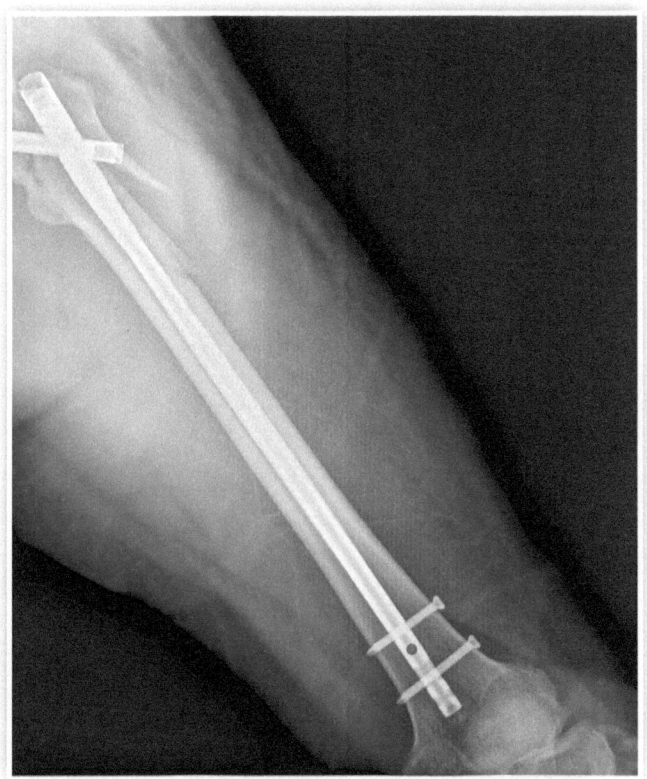

That is usually sufficient; but on some occasions, it is necessary to perform an initial open reduction of the fracture with ancillary use of cerclage wires, clamps or clips. These enveloping devices, alone, will not provide sufficient skeletal stability until union occurs. Instead, they can be a supplement to the attaining and maintaining of an anatomic reduction. Thereafter, a surgeon can rely upon the interlocked intramedullary nail for greater mechanical stability until union occurs.

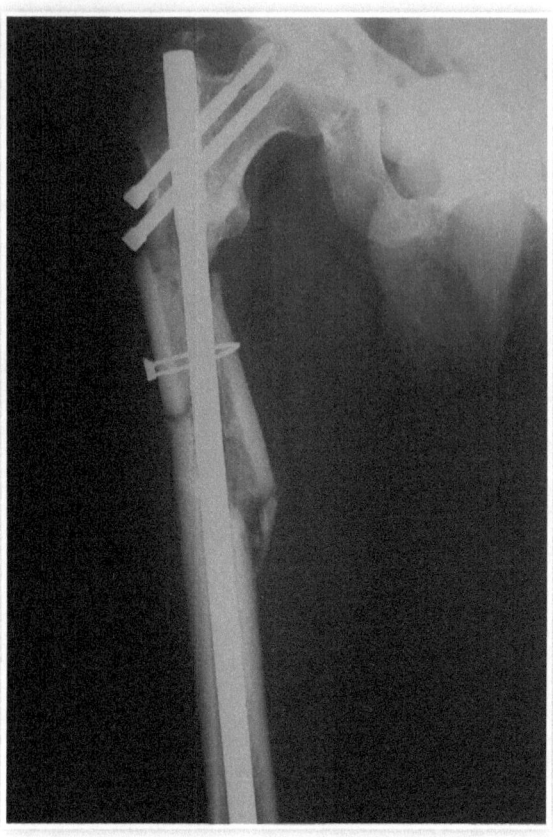

If these cerclage wires were not used, and significant displacement of a long spiral fracture persisted, the time to union could be two or three times normal. On average, most femoral fractures will unite within four to six months. In this hypothetical case, it might take eighteen months before the radiographs indicate that union had occurred.

Wishing to sue an operating surgeon for the attendant social, recreational and remunerative losses attendant on his failure to use the cerclage devices per operatively, the patient might approach the Office of the Health Ombudsman for some support. Usually, none is received. The Ombudsman might refer the matter to the State Medical Board, but the notification committees are usually similarly unimpressed. The test in negligence in law is whether the action of the operating surgeon was within the bounds of skill accepted by a significant body of colleagues then currently practising. This is sometimes referred to as the modified Bolam principle in Australian law. Other countries will have similar thresholds.

On this issue, opinion is divided. Some would have used some form of cerclage device. A reasonable number of others would have elected not to do so. Consequently, success with civil litigation was unlikely.

It is an unfortunate fact that some femoral fractures can take a long while to heal, which is why such matters are spoken of in averages.

GENERAL ADVICE

The Confounding Effects Of Time

Younger patients who have not yet reached skeletal maturity might be subjected to a constellation of quite severe and widespread injuries.

When a seven years old girl was struck by a motor vehicle, the force came from her right. She sustained a fracture of her clavicle, a fracture-dislocation of her shoulder, a fracture of her upper arm bone (the humerus), a dislocation of her elbow, and fractures of both forearm bones (the radius and the ulna). She had multiple rib fractures with an underlying pneumothorax requiring ventilation in an intensive care unit for nearly three weeks. She had closed pelvic fractures, a compound fracture of the thigh bone (the femur), and compound fractures of both shin bones (the tibia and the fibula). So severe were her injuries that she required seven operations, was hospitalised for a little over three months and lost one year of primary schooling. She was quite significantly disfigured from lacerations other than those associated with the operative scarring from her therapeutic regimen.

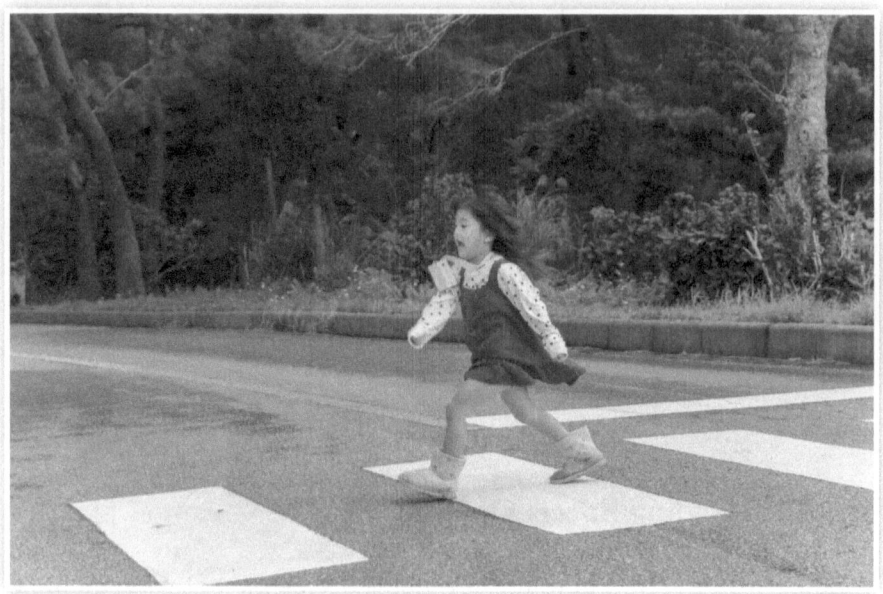

Fourteen years later, all her fractures had united, every joint had regained a full range of motion, there was no evidence of neurological sequelae, motor function was restored, there was no residual muscle wasting and no evidence of peri-articular or intra-articular instability. Apart from her scarring, she had made a complete recovery.

On measurement of her impairment because of her orthopaedic injuries, nothing could be quantified using the relevant chapters of the AMA 5 Guides. The only losses that could be quantified were those related to scarring, and these were best dealt with by using Chapter 8. Her parents and her solicitor were dismayed by a 0% orthopaedic impairment rating. It also surprised her medicolegal reporter, but it was the fact The Guides allow no room for emotion. Nor can they be manipulated through sympathy.

The effects of time can be quite extraordinary. *Tempus, edax rerum.* If only every outcome were so positive!

25

LEAD ARTICLE

Is The Insurer's Medical Expert In The Insurers' Pocket?

A loaded question obviously! It refers to medical experts who tend to identify with insurers, which are almost always in the camp of the insured defendants, rather than with plaintiffs.

Friendship is a very useful facility and one to be encouraged in our society. It permeates social, recreational and professional liaisons. It does not necessarily spell conflict of interest, nor should it be viewed as a threat. It should not lead a medicolegal reporter who is engaged by one side or the other to favour one over another when providing advice in litigation.

The unspoken premise of the rhetorical question here is that doctors who are "WorkCover friendly" are hard-nosed, disgruntled, suspicious and draconian; that they tend automatically to doubt the veracity of claims of injured plaintiffs, to take a purist's view of injury patterns, to fail to recognise that the spectrum of response to injury can be broad, and to distil every claim as they would to the lowest common denominator. It may be true that some practitioners who are highly competent at their work may have personality problems, either by natural or acquired character or as the result of current circumstances. They are all human, and in any case, their task is to give the patient the benefit of a competent report rather than to be a friend. Nevertheless, simple, straightforward, and sometimes hard statements of fact can leave an injured plaintiff bewildered. A courteous explanation can go a long way to defusing anger and frustration.

Statutory entities must operate within rules and guidelines. Injury scales are often proscriptive and prescriptive. They mandate the bases for assessment, and are there for all to see, to conform to, and to use against an expert who tries to evade the rules. Unlike the common law relating to compensation for personal injury, most Workers' Compensation Acts do not always recognise variations from the mean. Nuances that are sensitive to individual suffering are lacking. This is a possible reason why Tribunal determinations should be open to judicial review.

The position is somewhat different in common law claims, some of which relating to work injuries are covered by the defendant's Workers' Compensation policy. In those cases, there are no such mandates, but the processes of common law actions provide an efficient sieve through which to test opinions given in medical reports.

It should not really matter whether a medicolegal reporter has a strong and friendly association with WorkCover or not. The reporter's obligation is for a combination of neutrality, objectivity, transparency, and clarity of thought. An absence of any of these qualities rapidly becomes apparent under testing in the witness box. Persistence in the flawed mode rapidly produces a reputation that reduces the value of the reporter's opinion, and of the reporter's value to the client. Further, competent lawyers for a party find no comfort whatever in acting on a defective report, which misleads them and often leads to the most unfortunate results. In one matter, during an adjournment immediately after a medical reporter's evidence, he said to counsel who called him, "Did I say what you wanted?" The cold reply was, "You were to say it as it was: all I wanted was for you to tell me what it was, first."

To perform to those qualities is not difficult, and most practitioners, particularly those of high station in their profession, conduct themselves in this respect with high values. Any attempt to influence them improperly would be met with the highest disapprobation. There are always experts and lawyers who will not act to the highest standards, but they are quickly known.

On the insurer's side, its business consists in paying money in suitable circumstances to protect its insured with indemnity against any payment that the insured is properly liable to make. Good insurance managers, and there are many, are reasonably cautious to avoid fraud against their company, but do not resent such an obligation when it is just and correct. They would not countenance any attempt to compromise a reporting expert by wrongful influence. Those who are practical know that by the engagement of experts who have a reputation for reliability and integrity, their part in any litigation will have respect, with suitable benefits.

In fairness, it must be recalled that while some experts are regularly engaged on behalf of insurers, the same dynamics apply in the case of experts who are regularly engaged by solicitors specialising in that legal business, and who predominantly act for plaintiffs. The same influences apply, much the same responses appear, and the same proprieties should apply on that side also.

CASE VIGNETTE

Not Everything Is As It Seems

Orthopaedic surgeons rely heavily upon radiographs to diagnose fractures. Fractures in themselves can be sub-classified in myriad ways. The word "fracture" refers to a discontinuity in the normal structure of a bone. Bones are living organs and have cortical (outer) and cancellous (inner) components.

Plane radiographs, being uniplanar, are two-dimensional representations of a three-dimensional happening. Considerable overlay will be present on their film, and an undisplaced, relatively minor fracture may not be visible on them initially. The scaphoid, one of the small bones in the wrist, is a classic example. It is about the size and shape of a cashew nut, and is vulnerable to fractures through its' "waist", or mid-section.

This is especially true in patients who have fallen on an outstretched hand or wrist. The patient will almost invariably complain of pain in the anatomical snuffbox, the small space just at the base of the thumb, but the initial x-ray or radiograph may not show anything untoward. Displaced fractures are relatively easy to identify on the radiograph. It is the initially undisplaced fracture that can troublesome.

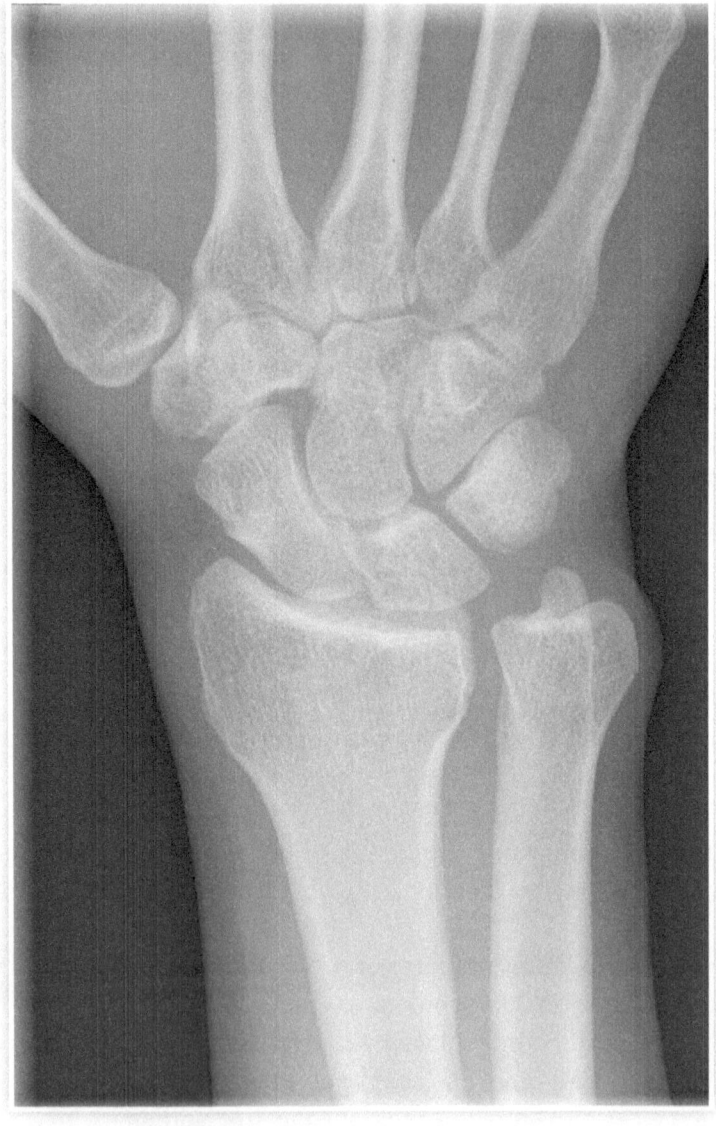

An undisplaced, barely visible fracture through the scaphoid "waist"

Part of the biology of fracture healing is initiated by hyperaemia, an increase in blood flow at the site. A secondary effect is for the radio-opaque minerals at the fracture edges to be resorbed. Once this process has been in train for ten to fourteen days, the mineral-leached fracture zone appears darker on a subsequent x-ray or radiograph. The diagnosis is then easier to make. As the healing process continues, new mineral is deposited, the area becomes more radio-opaque or white, and the diagnosis is equally obvious.

It is this difficulty in diagnosis of the initially undisplaced fracture that interferes with management decisions.

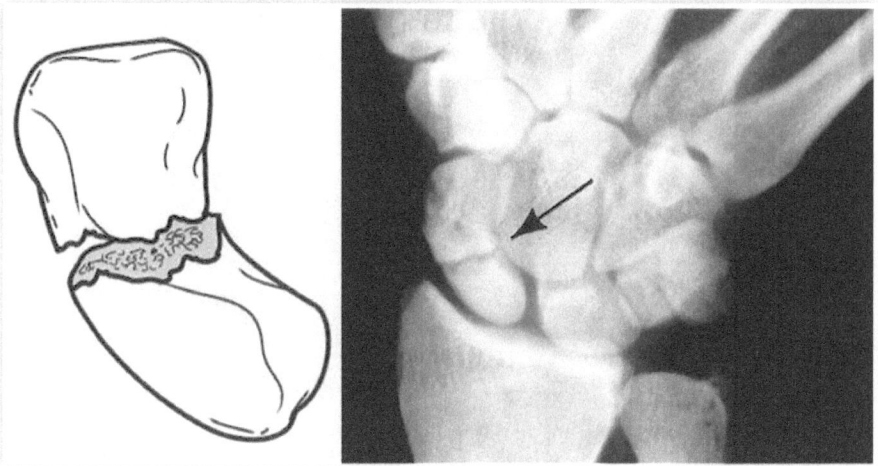

The fracture has not healed. The proximal pole is dead (dense or white)

The correct approach is to have a high index of clinical suspicion. If the patient has a history of having fallen on an outstretched hand or wrist, and has considerable pain localised to the anatomical snuffbox and yet has a normal radiograph, it is prudent to immobilise the wrist as though a scaphoid fracture was present. The cast can then be removed two weeks later, a new radiograph performed, and the underlying presence of a scaphoid fracture can then either be confirmed or excluded.

Failure to adopt this suspicion at the beginning, and a further consequent failure to immobilise the wrist immediately, would increase the risk of delayed or non-union. The blood supply (and therefore the supply of healing nutrients) to the scaphoid is from distal to proximal. The proximal pole of the scaphoid is at risk of death due to avascularity. The risk is potentiated by excessive movement at the fracture site during the healing phase. Its ramifications can be dire, consisting at least of prolonged pain, disability, incapacity and ongoing medical costs.

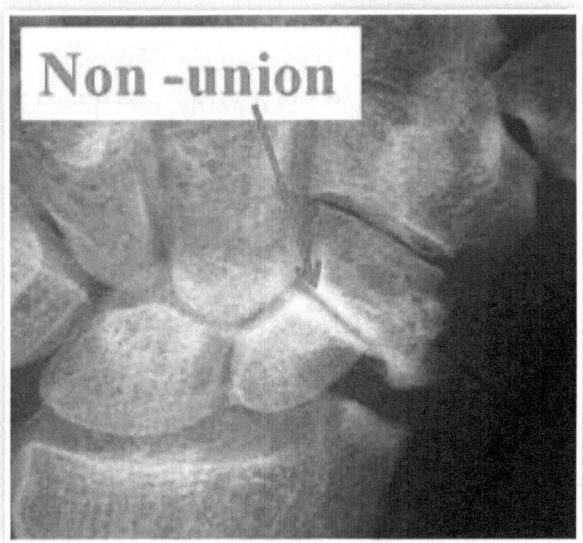

Established non-union with sclerotic (white) margins

So well understood and widely known is this potential problem that in the event of such failure, a claim of negligence would be difficult to defend.

GENERAL ADVICE

Is The Expert Suitably Qualified?

The topic of experts' straying beyond their field of expertise has already been discussed. A different paradigm relates to the need of experts for some form of certification or qualification according to a jurisdiction or legislation. For example, Workers' Compensation insurers require that, to be engaged by them, expert reporters are familiar with their specific requirements. Initial registration requires some form of validation of competence. Training courses are mandated. They include course work and examinations. Recertification is also expected periodically.

The American Medical Association publishes the "Guides to the Evaluation of Permanent Impairment". It is in the sixth edition. Some jurisdictions insist upon AMA 4, AMA 5 or AMA 6. It is imperative that a medical expert reporter has been both trained in the relevant module and has current certification that the training has been completed.

Without these respectively relevant qualifications, an expert's report might be rejected. The answer is to ensure in advance that the expert engaged is qualified for the particular task in the jurisdiction.

LEAD ARTICLE

When Is Apportionment Appropriate?

Is the clinical condition displayed by a plaintiff following an injury due in its entirety to the injury? Stated differently, "not all damaged goods were pristine prior to the subject accident".

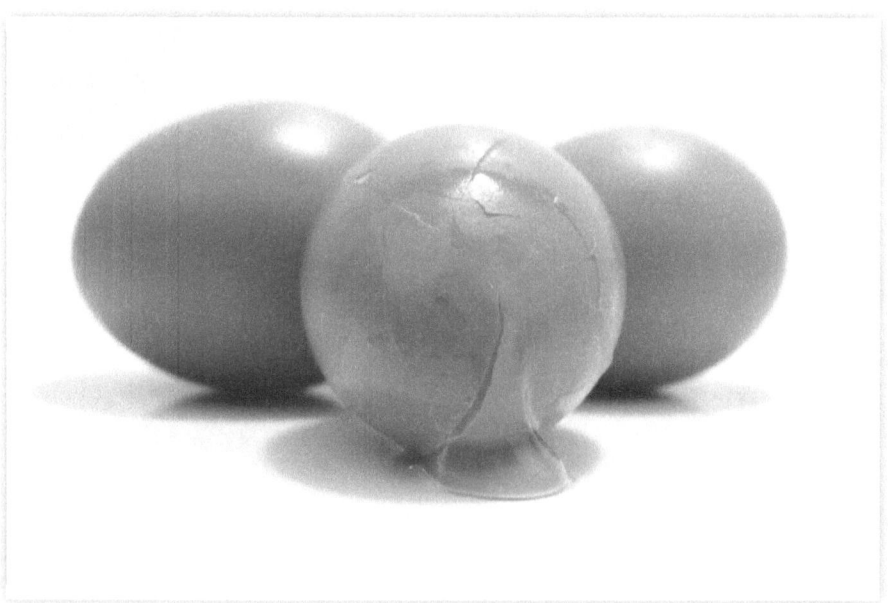

It is suitable for this discussion to focus upon a lumbar spinal injury suffered by two different hypothetical plaintiffs.

Plaintiff A is a sixty-three year old lady who gave a history of thirty years of prior back pain. She had undergone two separate operative procedures, the last of which was 18 years before the relevant accident. During the prior ten-year period before it, and despite her long history, she had been functioning relatively well, working full-time, playing bowls and golf and some social tennis.

Her relevant injury occurred at her supermarket workplace as she was leaving its cold room. Her arms were laden with stock replenishments. She slipped on a pool of water, fell heavily onto her bottom, and sustained a serious crush fracture of L3. She did not require operative intervention, but hospitalisation was part of her therapeutic programme. She wore a brace for nearly three months. With the combination of physiotherapy, rehabilitation, hard work and determination, she regained some semblance of her former life.

On assessment for medicolegal purposes, it was found that she had a loss of 20% of whole person function, which translated indirectly to significant disabilities at social, recreational, domestic and remunerative levels. Several experts opined that, had she been assessed critically and objectively immediately prior to this fall, she would have been experiencing a loss of 15% of whole person function. The Court determined therefore that this additional loss of 5% of whole person function was the compensable part.

The **second Plaintiff**, also female, but only twenty-four years of age, categorically denied previous problems referable to her lumbar spine. She had never experienced pain, stiffness or a work injury. There had been no prior work loss, chiropractic treatment, physiotherapeutic intervention, radiographic examination or any other problem referable to her lumbar spine.

In the course of her work, she was assisting a fellow worker to lift a very heavy object, and felt something "unusual" in her lumbar spine. Over the next few hours, that sensation became quite painful, and within two or three days, she had leg pain and numbness consistent with sciatica. Careful examination and investigation confirmed that her L5/S1 disc was anomalous. Its nucleus was protruding so that it was compromising her spinal canal and her exit foramen. Impingement upon her left S1 nerve root explained her sciatica.

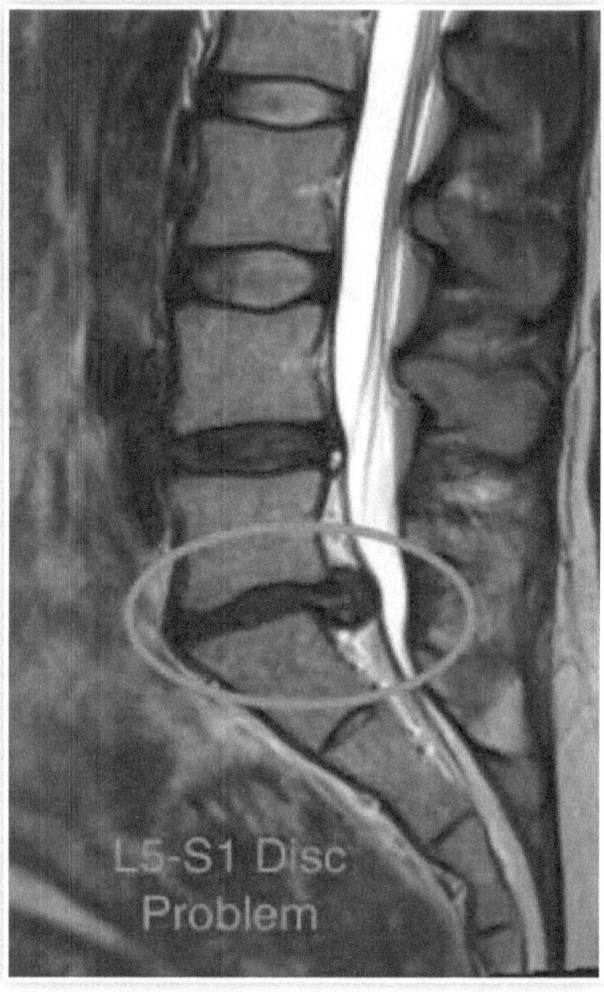

The ruptured disc is protruding rearwards and compromising the cauda equina

When her case came to trial, the experts generally agreed that her L5/S1 intervertebral disc had been degenerate prior to her relevant injury, since an MRI scan examination conducted soon after it confirmed that the disc was already abnormal. However, several of them agreed that, had it not been for the imposition of this particular force, she may have continued to have been asymptomatic indefinitely, without ever being aware that the disc was diseased. MRI scan examinations that reveal abnormal discs are very common, even in people in their twenties and thirties. Most of them are unaware of the abnormality, and some might remain pain-free for the remainders of their lives.

This plaintiff was assessed as suffering a 6% whole person impairment according to the AMA 5 Guides. Although the disc was probably degenerate prior to the accident, her entire loss was held to have been attributable to the lifting incident. No apportionment was necessary.

Why So Different?

The most significant difference between these patients is age. The first lady was sixty-three years of age whereas the second lady was only twenty-four years. Other subtle differences maybe related in part to that factor. The first gave a long history of discomfort: the second had no such history and despite rigorous scrutiny of her clinical records, no contradictory evidence was ever found. Other differentiating factors include the first patient's having undergone surgical procedures whereas the second had not. With the first, her fall created a new, and easily recognisable crush fracture of a vertebral body. With the second, the depredations to the disc were partly new and partly old.

In essence, there is no single specific rule as to whether apportionment is necessary or not. Whether apportionment is appropriate will depend on all the vagaries involved and is best applied on a case-by-case basis. Importantly, the reasons for or against any apportionment must be provided as part of the opinion. It is ultimately for the Court to decide the issue.

CASE VIGNETTE

Lovers' Heels

"Lover's heels" refers to fractures of one or both calcanei or heel bones. It is classically sustained by a male who has been unexpectedly found in a bedroom with another man's wife. As the husband ascends the steps to the bedroom, the lover jumps from the bed, runs to the verandah, and leaps over the railing. His landing on the concrete driveway three metres below gives rise to this most unpleasant injury. Men who might find themselves in this causal situation should avoid it altogether; but if the primary attraction is insuperable, stay in bed and face the music. It is likely to be less painful than a calcaneal fracture. Of course, not all such injuries are the result of such antics.

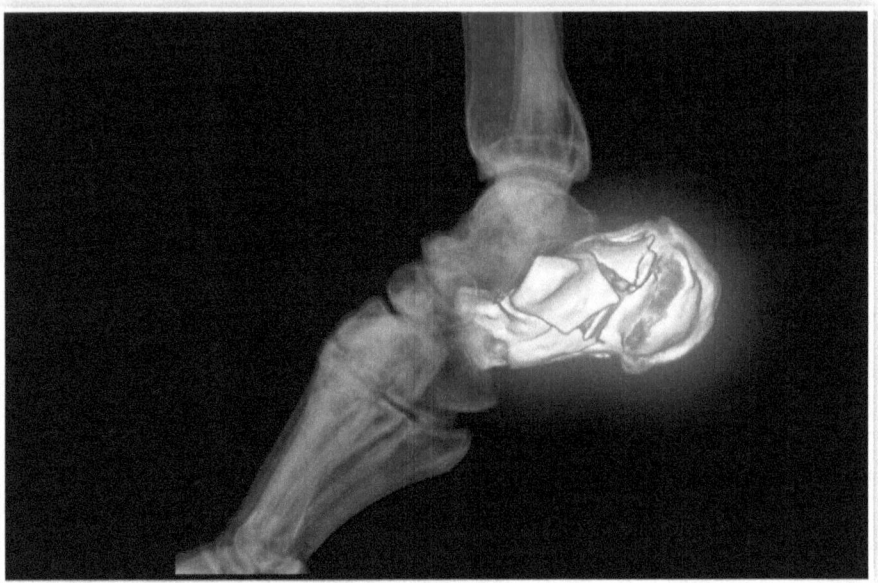

Grossly comminuted heel fracture

Heel fractures can be particularly troublesome. They give rise to extreme pain and extraordinary swelling, for which, bed rest, elevation, ice and analgesia are the hallmarks of early treatment. This is especially true if the fracture is extensive and comminuted, that is, having many fragments.

The calcaneus contributes to a very important joint with the ankle bone, or talus. This subtalar joint allows the heel to move inwards and outwards when walking over uneven terrain. If this movement is restricted because of post-traumatic arthritis, walking becomes particularly arduous and almost impossible on soft sand or construction sites, or through rough bush.

Calcaneal fractures can also be managed surgically. The procedure may require a piecing of the small fragments together, a little like the unsuccessful surgery on Humpty Dumpty. They can be held in position with plates, screws, wires and other devices. Nonetheless, the joint between the talus and the calcaneus is often irreparable.

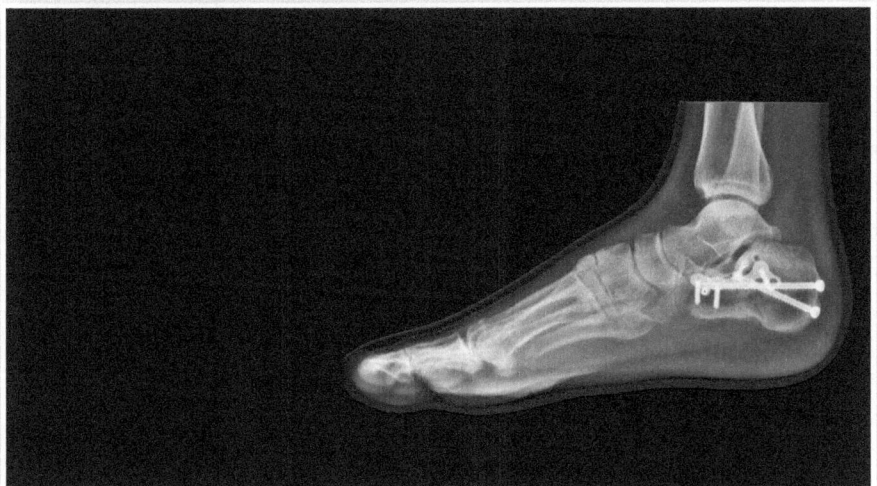

This calcaneal fracture has been internally fixed

An alternative salvage operation takes the form of a subtalar fusion, an arthrodesis. It is very useful, since it can convert a stiffish, painful joint into a stiff, painless joint. The patient loses about 10° of inversion and eversion of the heel, but also loses the pain, a most attractive trade-off.

GENERAL ADVICE

Complex Injuries In Complex Patients

A lady was born with phocomelia, affecting her left upper limb. Her major arm bone, the humerus, was congenitally absent. This is obviously a serious physical disability, but she had learnt adaptive procedures that rendered her independent and employable.

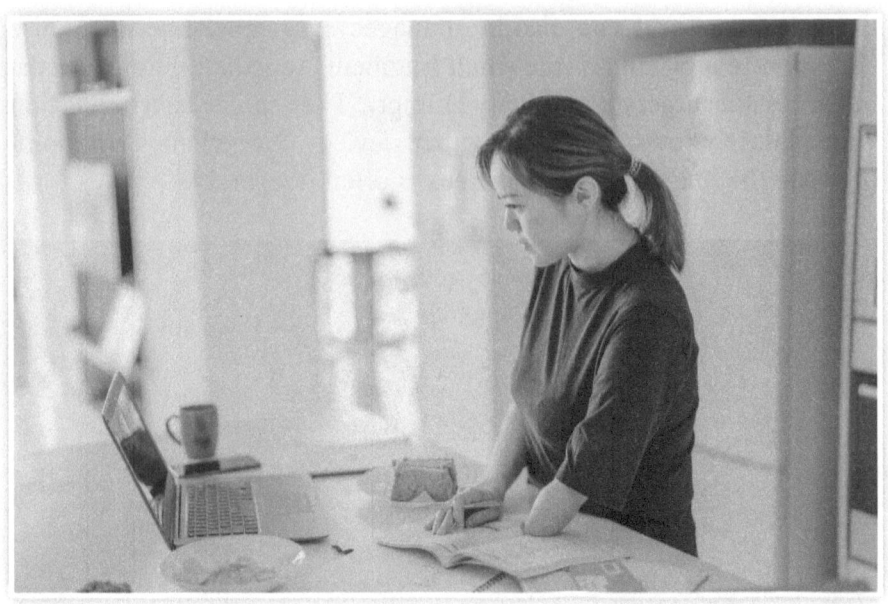

Although young, she was divorced and provided care for her dependent four-year-old son. Special ergonomic workplace modifications allowed her to be gainfully employed in a small electric-engine factory. A sling device was attached to her shortened left upper limb allowing her to stabilise an object on her work bench. Her right-hand dexterity was almost miraculous and she could use all manner of tools to accomplish her tasks. She then suffered a serious crushing injury to this important right hand. Despite complex hand surgery and extensive rehabilitation, she could not return to her former employment, for her congenital deficiency added materially to her eventual disability.

From a medicolegal perspective, her general damages would be the same as those of a normal person. Remunerative losses were another matter. A wrongdoer takes the victim as he finds him, or her, so that the loss is measured only by the difference between what is and what would have been. A vulnerable plaintiff's damages are diminished only to the extent of an allowance for any probability that the vulnerability may have led in some way to a diminution of future loss. This lady's future economic loss was significant. Whereas another worker may have been able to re-enter the workforce, albeit at a lower level of remuneration, her future remunerative prospects had been extinguished. The only issue was the amount of the allowance to be made for the risk that, if she had not so been injured, some future event might affect her earning capacity. That exercise would consider the risk that her prior vulnerability may have perpetuated that result.

This differs from a discount of measurable residual impairment and disability because of pre-existent maladies, and the apportionment that might ensue.

27

LEAD ARTICLE

How Much Explanation Is Too Much?

We can agree that the AMA (5) Guides are both prescriptive and proscriptive. Table 17.2 is a perfect example. When assessing a lower limb impairment, there is a serious risk of measuring the same functional loss more than once, and summating them in a simple arithmetic addition, rather than allowing for overlap. Muscle weakness and wasting have different parameters, with different impairment tables, but they emanate from the same loss, and act together. Similarly, a joint with severe arthritis pain will invariably have restricted ranges of movement and it would be inappropriate to summate or combine both.

Trained AMA 5 experts should be skilled assessors of musculoskeletal disease. They must perform precise and accurate examinations and translate this information into a final measurement of whole person loss (or % impairment) by interpreting the Guides appropriately. Whilst the methodology used can be open to question under cross-examination, detailed descriptions of the processes involved do not necessarily need to be incorporated into the expert's report to the Court.

An undesirable approach is to tediously quote the Guides, explaining every step in the process of quantifying an impairment. With plaintiffs suffering numerous injuries, this could add several pages of typed text to a report.

Alternatively

A more succinct analysis could be that, *"The plaintiff has suffered extremely severe injuries to the affected lower limb, involving skeletal, muscle and peripheral nerve losses. He has now reached a state of maximal medical improvement (MMI) and can be accurately assessed according to the AMA (5) Guides. Whilst his deficits include muscle weakness and wasting, difficulties with ambulation, pain and discomfort, the need to use a cane for support, and similar related maladies, he is best assessed using Table 17.33 to allocate a loss of 20% of lower extremity function because of his fractures, and a further loss of 66% of lower extremity function because of his neural injuries. When these two losses are combined using Combined Values Tables, a loss of 74% of lower extremity function can be quantified. This equates to a loss of 29% of whole person function".* Understand that considerable time and effort underpin this distillate. The precise workings can be explored under cross-examination is necessary.

In Summary

Less can be both useful and enough, and it may contribute to clarity by avoiding the pitfall of distraction, both in the writing and in the reading. Challenge the expert if the assessment seems incongruous or departs significantly from the norm established by other reporters. In essence though, more is not necessarily better.

CASE VIGNETTE

Not All Prior Injuries Remain Relevant

A 38-year-old male motorcyclist, who had never been in paid employment, sustained a fracture involving the upper end of his shin bone (the tibia), in an accident about twenty years previously. His injury required open reduction and internal fixation with a plate and screws. Despite valiant efforts on the part of the surgeon, only an incongruous or uneven joint surface was achieved. He was destined to suffer with osteoarthritis in his knee joint at some time in the next twenty, thirty or even forty years. The original metalware was removed when he was in his late twenties.

Quite recently, he had another motorcycle accident, resulting in severe fractures to the lower end of his thigh bone (the femur), which formed the knee joint with that same, previously injured shin bone. Although metal plates and screws were inserted in the femur, it was simply impossible to reconstruct his knee joint. The fractures united and the joint remained stable, but it could barely bend, was constantly swollen, and remains extremely painful. It is typical of end-stage osteoarthritis.

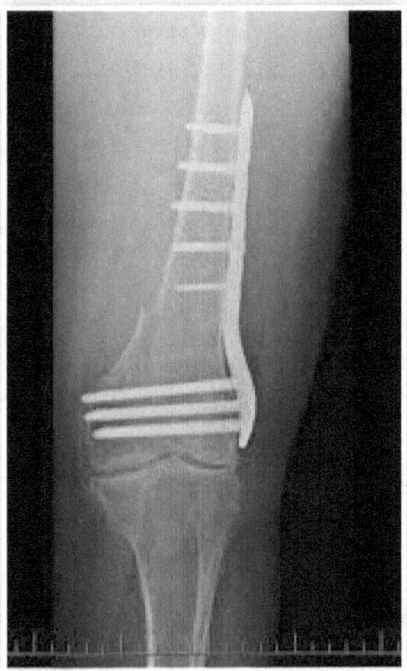

*The femoral fracture has been internally fixed.
The joint remains arthritic.*

Despite his relative youthfulness, he would benefit most from a total knee replacement, a very major undertaking in a young man. If he was to live until his mid-eighties, which, of course, depends upon his no longer motorcycling, he will likely require one total knee replacement, will have a 50% chance of requiring a second one (a revision), and about a 10% chance of requiring a further one (a re-revision). Extraordinary costs would be involved, as well as a plethora of possible complications.

It would be reasonable for the Defendant to a claim in respect of the more recent accident to argue that he would already have required a total knee replacement at some time in the future, even if this more recent accident had not occurred. Though that is true, the adverse effects of the prior accident will have been grossly overshadowed by the severity of this most recent injury to such magnitude that the original injury of two decades ago is probably no longer of any relevance. Even in the absence of the first accident, the adverse effects of this subsequent accident possess the ability to create the proposed scenario.

This would be an important issue to be addressed by the Court. There would be questions as to how apportionment can be calculated accurately, whether his history is relevant, and whether and to what extent in these circumstances, the defendant was obliged to accept the plaintiff as he found him. Clearly, these complex issues are beyond the province of the medical expert.

GENERAL ADVICE

How Can We Share Knowledge?

Continuing Professional Development (CPD) is both vital for our performance and mandatory for our registration.

The basic principle is derived from the value of the acquisition of concurrent knowledge and the ability to use it wisely. Practitioners can read journals, undertake research, attend conferences, participate in workshops, or engage in peer-reviewed activities. All modalities have their place, but a two-way exchange may well be the most valuable. There is undoubted value in attending a conference for six or seven hours a day, for three days, in a distant city, but it somewhat loses its charm in the atmosphere of dimmed lights, monotonous tones of the speakers, and when the late nights beforehand are all particularly soporific. In a workshop environment however, and with relatively small numbers, the participants are more likely to remain awake and alert, will have a higher degree of focus, and can both receive and offer ideas of interest. The experience will be active rather than passive.

At a workshop at an inner-city hotel in New York, organised by one of the larger legal firms in the USA and with a national footprint, there were three speakers. The topic was particularly interesting, "The assessment of complex injuries in complex patients", and there was ample opportunity for two-way exchange over a delicious breakfast. Because it was a relatively early-morning event, most brains were clear, a finite end point to the meeting was defined, and circumlocution was eliminated. It was an extremely valuable and instructive ninety minutes.

Maybe we should do this more often?

LEAD ARTICLE

When Pain Is A Pain

Pain is the predominant symptom in 95% or more of orthopaedic conditions. Patients rarely complain of deformity, functional loss or malalignment. The presenting complaint is almost always of pain.

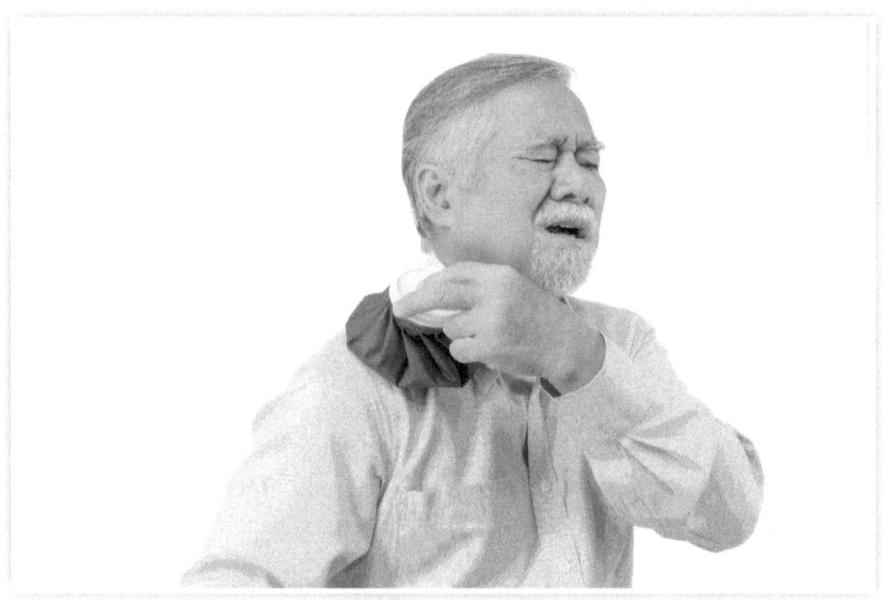

The word, "pain", can be defined in several ways. It is generally agreed that it is a highly unpleasant physical sensation caused by illness or injury. In that sense, the word is being used as a noun. It can also be used as a noun in a different mode. For example, "She took pains to see that everyone ate well". That means only she took the trouble or expended the necessary effort. The word can also be used as a verb. For example, "It pains me to say this", where the word is being used metaphorically rather than literally.

With the frequency of a complaint of pain in the symptomatic presentation of patients, it must be taken seriously. As clinicians, we are interested in many of its facets. Especially its nature and intensity, when it began and ceased, exactly where it is located, its duration and frequency, aggravating factors that may influence it, and relieving factors. A skilled clinician will elicit sufficient detail concerning all those variables so that in 85% of cases, a diagnosis could reasonably accurately be made before touching the patient. The physical examination, and the use of ancillary investigations, improves the diagnostic accuracy to approximately 99%.

Despite efforts expended in attaining precision in analysing pain, a medical expert must also deal with perceptive variables. Some patients describe a pain as almost intolerable, as though someone was poking a sharp knife through their eye, though their actual knowledge of that experience must be doubted. Others take pride in claiming that they "have a high pain threshold", though generally, almost always, they have a threshold far from high.

For impairment assessments, medical experts use texts such as the American Medical Association publication entitled "Guides to the Evaluation of Permanent Impairment" (5th Edition) as their reference. Functional losses, expressed as percentages of the whole person, usually relate to specific diagnoses or restrictions in range of motion of a joint or dysfunctions of a nerve. The pain factor, of itself, does not contribute greatly to this overall picture. Chapter 18 deals with it specifically but allows no more than a maximum of 3% whole person impairment. This is because all the other tables and figures in the AMA5 Guides consider, not only the diagnoses or functional limitations, but subliminally include pain as part of the presenting malady.

Medical experts separate symptoms from signs and subdivide findings into objective and subjective categories. For example, a patient with muscle wasting in the thigh or a swollen knee joint can be assumed to be suffering with some problem. It is difficult to pretend either or both clinical signs as they are objective manifestations of a clinical condition. Conversely, pain of which a plaintiff complains is difficult to confirm or quantify. It is this subjective component that leaves the authors of the AMA5 Guides little choice but to place impairment emphasis elsewhere. The AMA5 Guides, in Chapter 18, clearly outline the circumstances where the additional 3% WPI, or part thereof, can be added.

CASE VIGNETTE

Military Service And Tribunal Claims

When attempting to link medical conditions with prior military service, the issue of causation can be particularly vexing. All too often, the nexus is quite nebulous. For example, a seventy-year-old male with exceedingly severe degeneration or spondylosis throughout his cervical spine, thoracic spine and lumbar spine would have much difficulty in convincing a Tribunal that his widespread disease is due to a single heavy bounce in an army tank during a training exercise forty-five years previously. Despite the obvious difficulty in these cases, the gap maybe bridged in suitable circumstances.

In establishing causation, several features may be very helpful. They can be summarized as follows:

1. A specific event

This refers to an injury or accident that occurred at a defined moment in an identifiable location, resulting in an obvious adverse outcome and leading to a recognised condition.

2. A temporal link

As the time from injury to the onset of symptoms increases, the existence of a causal link become more tenuous. If the claimant in the army tank accident mentioned above had immediately complained of pain, had it recorded, and exhibited an unbroken link of symptoms between the event and his current claim, causation would be more confidently accepted.

3. Adequate investigation and the making of a diagnosis

Rather than in respect of some injury that had never been complained of or investigated and diagnosed over a lengthy period, the circumstances of a claimant's presenting, with clear investigation results performed in a timely manner confirming the diagnosis, again supports the likelihood of a causal link.

4. Operative intervention

If the injury or insult is of such severity that operative intervention was required immediately or soon thereafter, or at least with a traceable link into the future, again, causation is more likely.

5. Adequate notations

The military claimant referred to above had not been consulting with a General Practitioner, had not undergone any other investigations as an interim measure, had not received any form of treatment and could not otherwise in any way reasonably link the distant event with his current presentation. But, if excellent notes had been made at the time, if he had been a regular attender with a practitioner who had also kept good records, if he had been subjected to reasonable and diagnostic investigations and followed an expected natural history, then his claim may have been more acceptable.

There is no crystal ball which guarantees accuracy. All that can be done is to estimate, interpolate and extrapolate. The more secure the evidence, the more likely it is that causation can be confirmed (or excluded).

GENERAL ADVICE

Are Surveillance Videos Worth Their Salt?

As the economy bites more deeply, as more spurious claims follow, and as insurers become wiser, so there is a greater number of surveillance videos forming part of briefs for a medical review. It is better to view the video before seeing the plaintiff. That allows the reporter to form some opinion about the claimant's physical capacity, and to pose direct questions or even perform specific tests to assess the accuracy of the performances on screen and in person.

In one case, a lady in her forties claimed that her state was so severe that she rarely left her wheelchair, let alone her place of residence. During the trial, defence counsel produced a contemporaneous video recording her water skiing. While that alone was memorable, the fact that she was topless made it indelible.

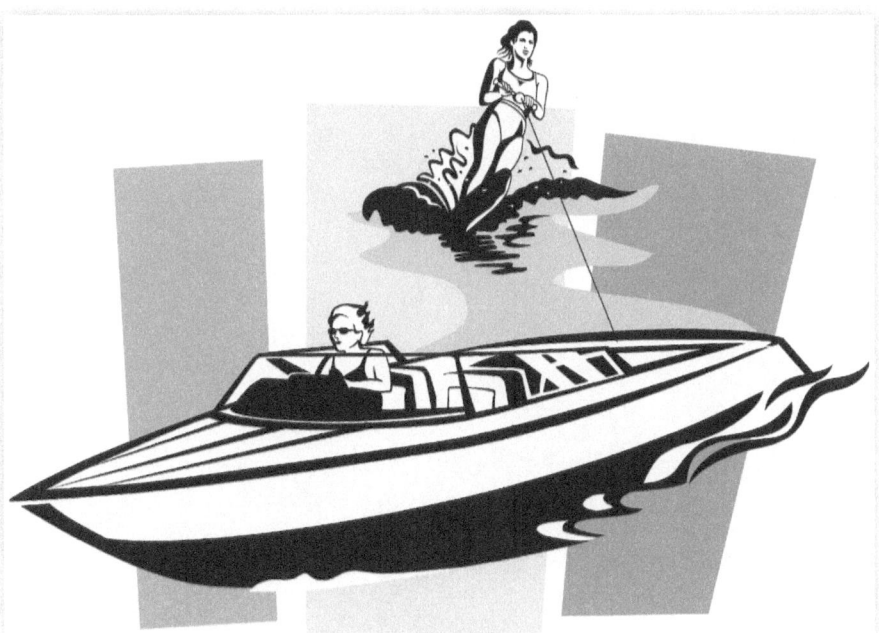

Such a dramatic exposé is unusual. More often, the evidence consists of grainy images where the subject is partially or completely obscured by vegetation, motor vehicles or buildings. Glimpses are brief, or the plaintiff is not doing anything spectacular, and the observation becomes essentially worthless.

The securing of surveillance video evidence is for the defendant's lawyers to decide. If it is provided, a reporter should view it. It is most desirable that it be contemporaneous, that it is taken on different days, weeks or months apart, in different environments, and with the plaintiff's performing contrasting tasks.

LEAD ARTICLE

Are Conclaves Valuable?

The word, "conclave", is derived from *"cum clave"*, which is Latin for "with a key". The term, "hot tub", comes from vernacular, meaning that special environment in the Court room with the Judge, legal counsel and experts. The heat presumably radiates from the bodies, is contained in that confined space, and is admixed with differences of opinion and anxiety. Obviously, this is not a meeting of Cardinals, prior to the puff of white smoke up the chimney in the Vatican.

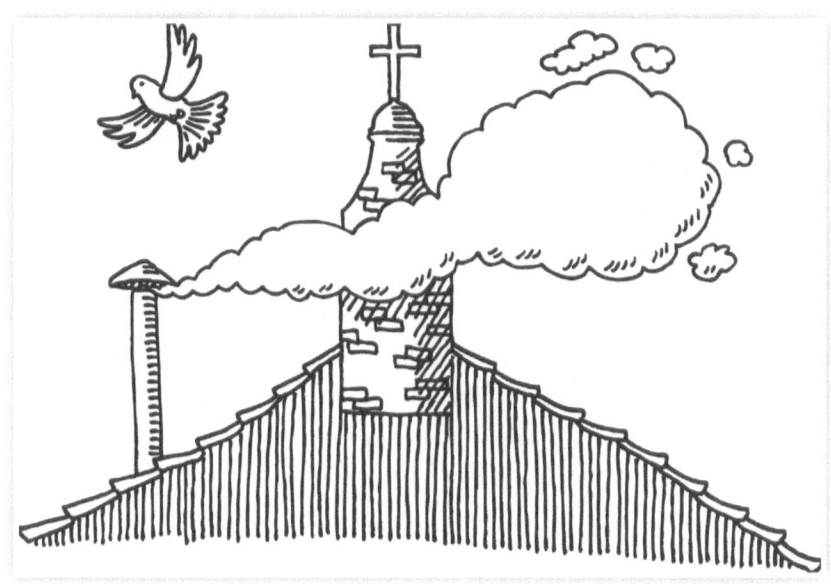

The concept of holding conclaves is not new. It dates back millennia and ancient tribes recognised the profits that could ensue. More recently, in the mid 1980's, the Federal Court in Australia came to adopt the concept, as did the Land Court. Such "hot tubbing" is a more recent arrival in Personal Injuries litigation. Its goal is to identify differences between experts, expose the reasons for them, fill any factual gaps, and then distil a unified opinion if possible.

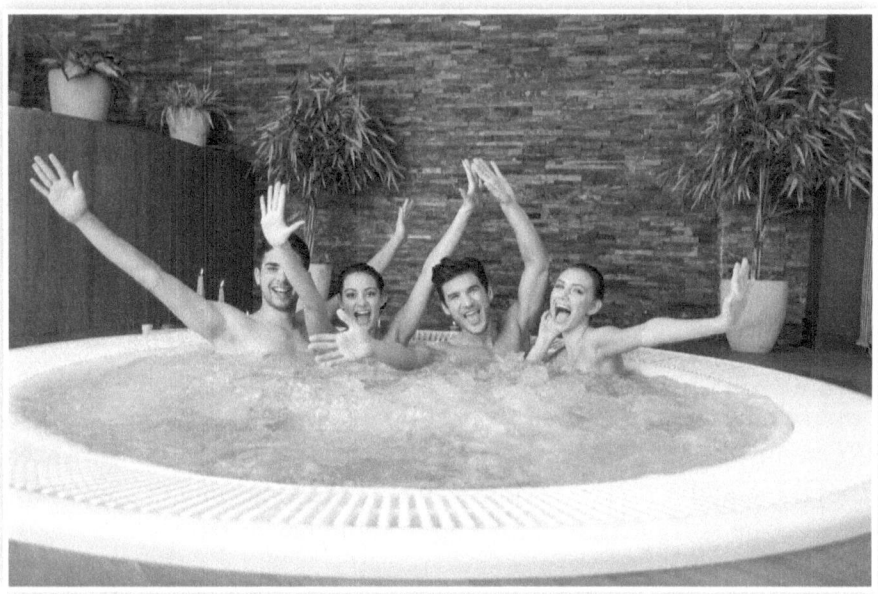

At first, this seemed to be avoidance of work by the Court, but it has proved to have great merit. The conclaves have been most enlightening, and often, the experts agree on most contentious issues. As for the few matters remaining, a brief discussion, the revelation of evidence of previously unrecognised facts or information, and a round-table chat, even one later on the telephone, can bring all to a satisfactory conclusion. The great benefits of course are the saving of Court time, the limiting of costs, the avoidance of the uncertainty of litigation, and the avoidance of unnecessary anguish for the litigious combatants.

CASE VIGNETTE

Even Santa Claus Is Vulnerable

Folklore has it that Santa became stuck in the chimney of an old house near the north pole years ago. There was no special obstruction in the chimney flue, but he was obese, his sack was heavily laden, and the bells on his waist became caught on the roughened interior. Fortunately, he could breathe, but his cries for help were muffed, and the terrified children who found him soon after dawn were understandably shocked. The Emergency Services team retrieved him and took him to the closest hospital. Radiographic examinations excluded any fractures, but his left lower limb had been caught in a fully flexed position so that the blood supply to the muscles below his knee had been seriously curtailed for more than four hours.

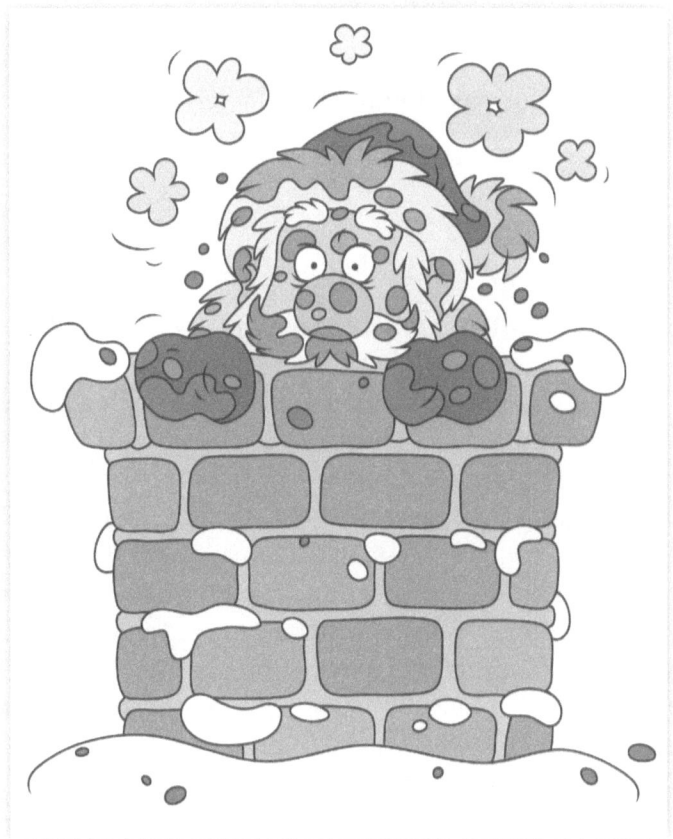

During Christmas Day, it became apparent that he had a compartment syndrome. Despite immediate decompressive fasciotomies, multiple operative procedures thereafter with skin grafting, and expert care, his limb was deemed to be non-salvageable. He was subjected to a below knee amputation in the third week of January. Though this type of case is rare enough to be worthy of a report, the scenario is quite well recognised. Inebriated revellers may fall asleep on a toilet, lie in remote locations without assistance, or be otherwise denied prompt therapeutic intervention, resulting in significant functional losses.

Because of the foreseeability of his entry by that means, and the householder's duty of care to make adequate provision for his safety in doing so, he was successful with his personal injury claim. This gave rise to the issue of damages, which in turn depended on the extent and nature of his loss through his injury. As early recognition of such an injury and prompt intervention become more common, these consequences will eventually disappear. And if Amazon takes over Santa's delivery role, with proper workplace health and safety initiatives, such occasions of injury may largely cease. Here come the drones!

GENERAL ADVICE

Who Oversees Medicolegal Report Quality Control?

It is difficult to know. In most countries, medical graduates are subject to registration requirements imposed by their national medical boards. Practitioners must register annually as it is not automatic, and there are hurdles to jump and hoops to pass through before registration is renewed. Continuing Professional Development (CPD) is part of the regimen. Those who undertake specialty programmes are vetted carefully and are often subjected to annual examinations. A final Fellowship examination is probably the most difficult exam that they will ever face, and this helps to ensure the quality of the service that they are providing.

All Members or Fellows of a College must remain current with CPD requirements. Random audits are undertaken and an entire College complement might be audited every five years. Subspecialty associations require members to undergo additional CPD training, which further ensures that they are remaining aware of current developments.

In the medicolegal arena however, entry is easy and free, so that there is no assurance that a medicolegal reporter is competent in the field. Though training programmes exist, attendance is not compulsory. Examinations are rarely set, and they are voluntary. The American Board of Independent Medical Examiners (ABIME) has a structured course programme, with examination for membership, but enrolment is again entirely voluntary. Many Australian medicolegal reporters continue to practice without visiting a single training session.

The effect on the quality of reports is obvious to practitioners in the field. Unsuspecting solicitors may not recognise a poor product, which can lead to unnecessary, lengthy and costly litigation, with a disappointing outcome.

It may be time to have an Australian College that exercises some control over the quality of the activity. Membership should be mandated, examinations set, and standards identified and maintained.

LEAD ARTICLE

How Unlucky Can You Be?

In a medicolegal examination for a workers' compensation insurer, the plaintiff, a gentleman who had been injured in a motor vehicle accident at work, was said to have sustained injury to his lumbar spine. Plane radiographic imaging confirmed that he had a prior problem with it, in the form of a forward slippage of one vertebral body on another. Such findings are not overly common in the lumbar spine, probably 4-5%, and not all of them are necessarily symptomatic. The condition is referred to as spondylolisthesis and comes in varying grades of severity.

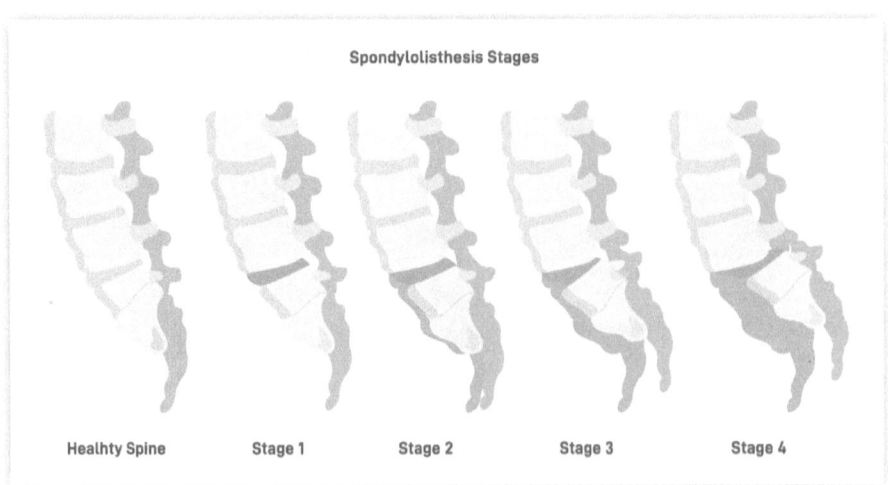

He had spent the preceding thirty years or so working in heavy laborious environments. It would have been unusual for one such as he to be truly asymptomatic prior to a potentially compensable road traffic accident. On close questioning as to prior back pain, stiffness, medical officer visits, radiographic examinations, employment related claims, visits to a chiropractor or a physiotherapist, and all other forms of possible indications of back symptoms, he was adamant in his denials, with assurances that his recent accident led to the beginning of his back problems.

The Sequence

Following this accident, he had been subjected to three separate operations and it was claimed that he was totally incapacitated for work. As he still had a couple of decades of potential working life, the size of the quantum claimed was considerably enlarged by this factor.

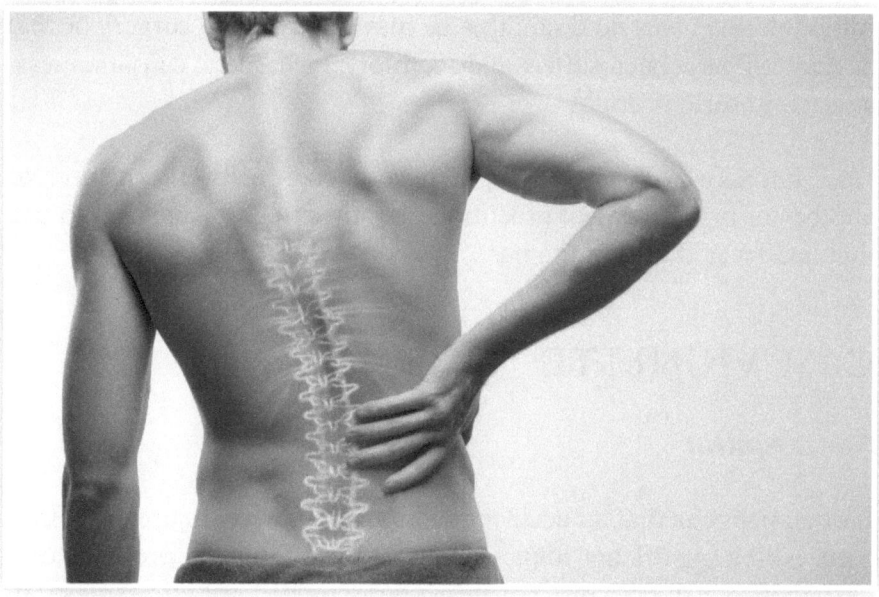

Though not doubting the accuracy of his denials, the medicolegal reporter took the precaution of referring in the report to the possibility that if the Court did not accept that he had been completely asymptomatic, any measurable functional impairment quantified in the report would be reduced, and an apportionment of blame might be appropriate, reducing his damages.

Oh Dear, You Guessed It ..

As fate would have it, the reporter's secretary, of the excellent memory, recognised the claimant's name, and a search of former records showed that he had consulted the reporter in the 1990's for clinical advice. He had been sent by a general surgeon who was concerned about his ongoing leg discomfort following an apparently successful hernia repair. He had presented with a history of back and leg pain. A radiographic examination had elicited a precise diagnosis of his spondylolisthesis – a quarter of a century before the subject accident.

It is probable that his symptoms referred to on presentation following his road traffic accident were related to his long-standing antecedent disease, so that any link with the claim accident became tenuous. Although there was no doubt that he may have needed surgery or that he may still have been suffering discomfort, the issue of causation was, at least, in serious doubt.

How unlucky he was! He might have been sent by the insurer to another of many medical practitioners rather than, by chance, to one that had treated him in the past.

CASE VIGNETTE

Non Sequitur

It often happens that an accident occurs, and a party injured in it may then exhibit significant impairments and loss. But the presence of a nexus between the two may not always be assured. The Latin expression, *"non sequitur"*, means that, in this case, the link of causation does in logic not necessarily follow. It is to be read with the expression, *"Post hoc, ergo, propter hoc"*, "after this, therefore, because of this", which is an expression used to exemplify a logical fallacy.

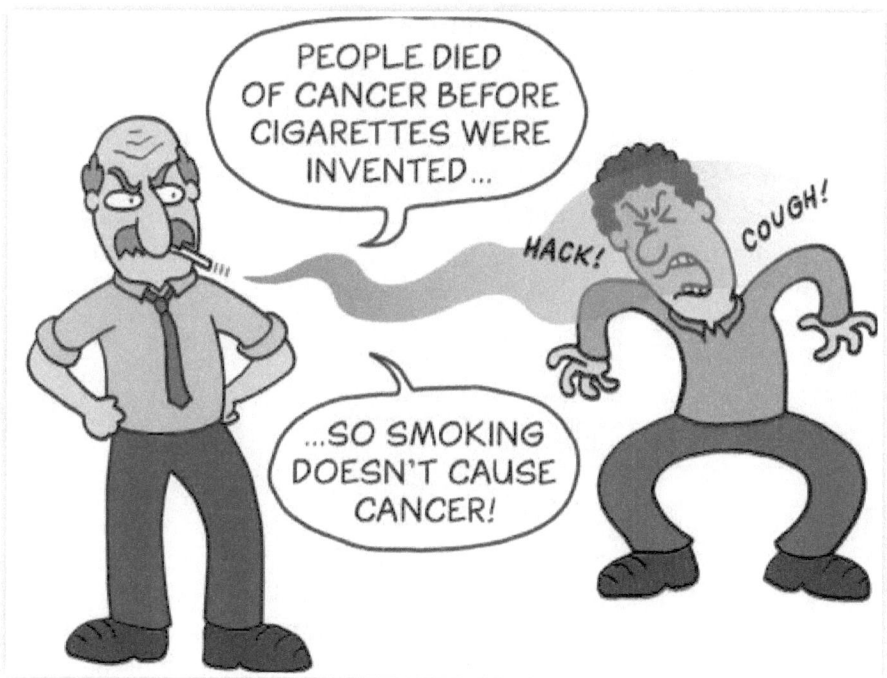

A 60-year-old male was a front-seat passenger in a motor vehicle, the driver of which turned right across the path of oncoming traffic. In the consequent collision, the force of the impact was heaviest on the patient's side of his vehicle and he sustained serious injuries. One related to his right knee. There was evidence of a direct blow over the front of his patella (kneecap), through contact with the dashboard. This knee had undergone an anterior cruciate ligament reconstruction twenty years previously. If he was to be believed, the reconstruction had been an outstanding success, and the joint had remained asymptomatic until the time of this accident.

It was clear that any functional loss that may have predated the accident was not linked with the accident, and conversely, there was some additional loss that could be linked with the accident. The blow to the patella had damaged the joint between the kneecap and the thigh bone, and that would have given rise to a measurable loss.

The defence argued to exclude any knee problem from the accident injuries because of this positive past history. The plaintiff opposed any exclusion or discounting for contribution. Common sense prevailed, a negotiated compromise reached, and fair compensation was paid.

The lesson is important, and sometimes overlooked. Damaged goods can be made worse. A pre-existent functional impairment can be aggravated, and significant additional impediments can accrue. It is through only a full history, a clinical examination, and a careful analysis that a true attribution and apportionment of blame can be identified.

GENERAL ADVICE

Talk, Talk, Talk

There is no property in a witness, which means that a witness must be free to be called by either side without hindrance by the other. Expert witnesses are within this principle, so that one side may call the other side's medicolegal reporter if that person's report is favourable to the party's case. That is an important reason why a reporter should be objective and non-partisan. The adversarial feature of law should be absent from medicolegal reports.

Medical experts however are humans, with emotions and opinions, and are sometimes biased, even sub-consciously, and regularly egocentric. Because an expert's primary duty is to assist the Court, a report prepared for it should exclude all these virtues. Perhaps they may be put to good use in a lawyer's seeking strategic advice from an expert, who may then approach the matter from that party's point of view, provided that there is no supply of material which is to be tendered in evidence. That activity might also exclude the expert's subsequently providing a report, but the advice given could be very useful at a litigious level.

How Might That Work?

If, for example, a lawyer has a client who is alleging negligence in the form of delayed emergency treatment at a hospital. A report from an interstate expert seems to support the claim, but another local expert, also engaged by the lawyer, expresses a contrary and adverse view in a report.

The truth may lie somewhere in between, and finding the most likely situation will become significant in deciding on the best strategy for the conduct of the claim. Identifying the strongest and most beneficial course can be very difficult without intimate knowledge of the clinical issue in question. This is where the strategic advisor could be of considerable advantage. Initially, by reviewing both opinions and identifying strengths and weaknesses on either side. Subsequently, by drawing the results together to advise the lawyer as to the most compelling answer, and perhaps to posit a case that, whilst not necessarily compelling enough for a Court, could substantially influence discussions during a mediation. It may not be successful, but it could assist the conduct of the plaintiff's claim and afford satisfaction in its assurance that the correct approach to the problem had been taken.

The same reasoning obtains if a similar problem was to confront a defendant.

This is an under-used process in the employment of expert advice and deserves more frequent consideration.

LEAD ARTICLE

Why Do Doctors Fear Litigation?

This discussion does not refer to doctors as expert witnesses. That can be stressful, though experience, proper preparation, and emotional disengagement usually dissipate any anxiety. Instead, it refers to a doctor's being sued.

Charges of unprofessional conduct and professional misconduct are usually dealt with by regulatory agencies. A civil claim for damages for negligence is often handled in civil jurisdictions of the Courts. The trial for a criminal offence is heard in a Criminal Court. The principles relating to claims for medical negligence are gathered in the modified Bolam standard which sets the threshold of acceptable medical conduct as one conforming to practices accepted by a cohort of peers as the usual test in Australia. Other countries have similar benchmarks.

For some medical practitioners, quite apart from any potential shame associated with being sued for professional negligence is the perception by some that justice is not always done to them, because of the restrictive rules applied by the Law. They feel that interpretations made by the Court may be unrealistic, unfair or plainly wrong. Counsel can be aggressive and particularly venomous, and the whole process may take many months or even years. These uncertainties generate great angst amongst them, but common sense would recommend an approach more philosophical and accepting of the process. However, fire does burn, and the scars are often permanent.

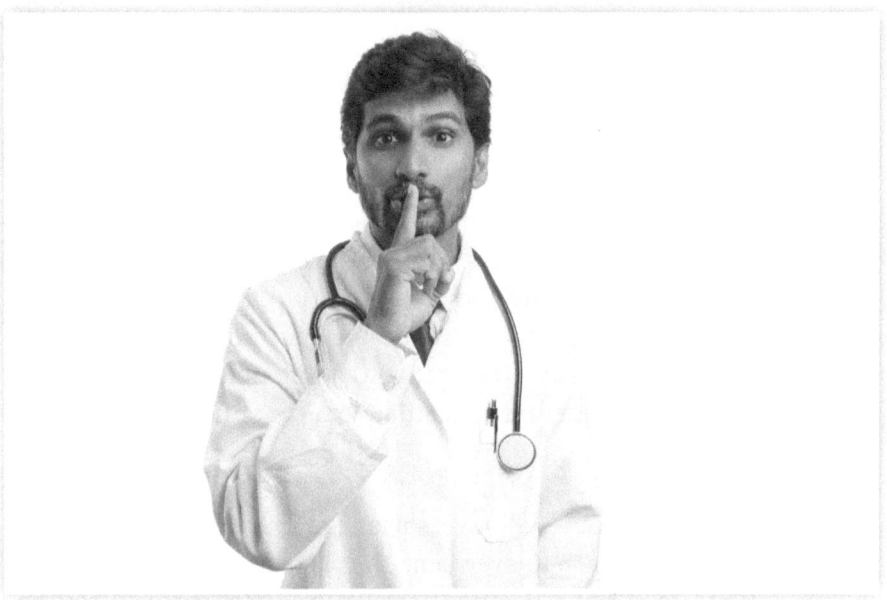

There are ways of diminishing the risk of litigation. Pre-emptive careful notetaking at the time of the conduct of the medical service, and establishing courteous rapport and remaining engaged at a professional level with potential claimants throughout the service usually pay dividends. They are not always effective in dissuading the commencement of an action, but if not, they may be useful in the defence, and the patient's attitude may be less antagonistic.

Medical defence organisations try to prepare their practitioners in a variety of ways. Emotional support is often provided and practitioners who are targeted should seek counsel and support from peers and professional organisations. Unfortunately, shame sometimes inhibits that type of openness and sharing, and the suffering is magnified.

There is no complete solution for the problem. There is fine synergy between the professions of law and medicine, and, despite the adversarial system, most lawyers accord medical practitioners against whom they are acting the courtesy of professional respect to the extent that it is appropriate.

CASE VIGNETTE

Indolent Infection Following Serious Injuries

Bacterial infections after trauma surgery continue to give rise to significant difficulties, whether it be in an emergency setting or at the time of an elective operation. The pivotal work of Fleming and Florey in bringing penicillin to market made an enormous change to the outcome of surgical activity. Research and development by major drug marketing companies has introduced a plethora of new and different types of antibiotics.

Unfortunately, their bacterial adversaries are extremely clever in the way they mutate and learn to overcome the obstacles presented to them by the antibiotics. They sometimes thrive in a post-surgical setting, despite reasonable efforts to defeat them. Some of the difficulty is of our own doing. Some practitioners use antibiotics unwisely, some patients do not always take a full course, and bacteria, whose virulence sets them apart in their ability to develop resistance, survive over antibiotic precaution. So serious is this problem that it is likely that infections could flourish in our own community because the bacteria achieve resistance to every chemotherapeutic agent available.

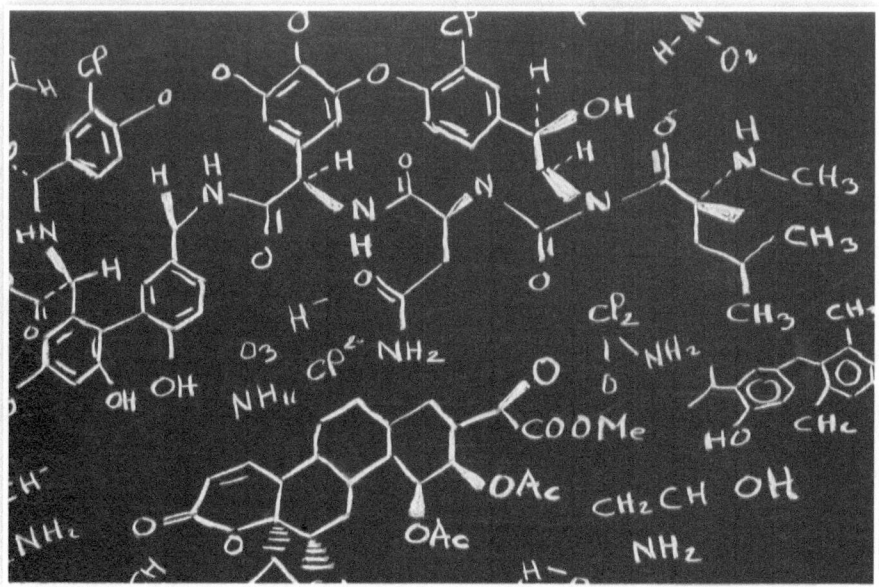

Most infections are obvious. They are accompanied by pain, redness, swelling, an increase in body temperature, and often a discharge of serous fluid or pus. Others, however, are vastly more subtle and can remain indolent for weeks, months, and even years. It is possible for an osteomyelitic bacterium to remain quiescent in a sequestrum (a small piece of dead bone in a parent bone) for some decades. It is only when that sequestrum or local deposit is disturbed, for example, at the time of an injury with a fracture, or at the time of a hip or knee replacement, that the bacterium is released and provoked into action with a spectacular infectious result.

Non-operative modalities such as the use of antibiotics are important in fighting infections, but it is the scalpel that is the most effective of all tools. Abscesses should be drained, dead and devitalised tissue debrided or removed, and vascularisation of the local region maximised. Received wisdom says, "heal with cold steel!"

The Relevance?

This has very special medicolegal implications. There is a risk that a patient may be deemed to have achieved the state of maximal medical improvement (MMI), where the condition could be thought to be both stable and stationary, and a claim could be closed prematurely. The recurrence of an indolent infection after claim closure could result in significant morbidity, great financial imposts, and even mortality. It is worthwhile to ensure that the medicolegal expert engaged considers this possibility when formulating a final report.

GENERAL ADVICE

Is There A Need To Standardise Personal Injury Claims Regulations?

Possibly. Australia is a good example. It covers an enormous area. Distances between cities are similar to those in the United States of America, though its population proportion is less than 10%. It has Federal laws governing many activities but there is significant duplication by State and Local Government regulations. The time may have come to standardise and unify those that apply to personal injury through negligence suits. An international approach could be even better.

Currently, some medical experts in one State are excluded from providing opinions in another State simply because they have not obtained the requisite certificates. The highest possible standards should be maintained, but reciprocity deserves consideration. It would avoid some duplication of effort, assist with a reduction in costs, and generally facilitate a smoother conduct of proceedings.

This is especially true in negligence cases. For valid reasons, Counsel may prefer to seek the advice of an expert from another State. This has the potential to diminish bias, improve objectivity, and avoid internal turf wars. Unless State barriers are reduced or removed, a quest for the ideal expert remains constrained.

A Tangential Thought

Some years ago, a Chief Justice of the Supreme Court, the Bar Association and the Law Society of a State declined to support a suggestion for the formation of a panel of experts to provide preliminary advice concerning the likelihood of success of the medical features in negligence cases on a *pro bono* basis. It seems that there can be many reasons, one of which could be the preservation of the Court's jurisdiction.

LEAD ARTICLE

How Important Is Empathy?

Vital! Medical experts are sometimes criticised for being harsh, aggressive, and wanting in the gentler emotions. Some of it is true. Their personalities are usually moulded well before doctors commence clinical practice, and little can be done to alter it. Nature and nurture have almost irreversible effects.

Plaintiffs who are attending for a medical assessment as a prelude to the preparation of a report for the Court are often unhappy, aggrieved, in pain, and anxious. Rage is almost palpable as some plaintiffs enter the consulting room. The practitioner's goal should be to have them leave in a calm, relaxed and contented mood. The practitioner's empathising with their circumstance is more than reasonable. In fact, it is probably mandatory as a matter of logical humanity, since the outcome of the issues is yet to be determined, and the expert may not be aware of all the evidence. Empathy is one of the many tools available to that end. Expressing sympathy, behaving courteously, and proceeding with care and compassion are all advisable.

Naturally, some caution should be exercised. It would be unwise to be seen as supportive of the plaintiff's claims. Empathy can be expressed without commenting upon liability, or the causation, nature and extent of the party's injuries.

CASE VIGNETTE

Past History Is So Very Important

A female patient was seriously injured in a road traffic accident whilst descending a mountain range on a very powerful Harley Davidson motorcycle. On assessment for the first time three years later, after she had reached maximal medical improvement (MMI), she had very severe muscle wasting of the left thigh. At a point 10cm above the superior pole of the patella, its girth was 4cm less than that of the right thigh. This was quite significant, given that she had a body mass index of only twenty-two. As she was relatively trim. her injured thigh was very skinny.

She had been categoric in her denials of prior problems referable to that thigh or of any problem in the region of the lumbar spine, her hip joint or her knee joint. In the absence of any evidence to the contrary her muscle wasting was believed to be wholly attributable to her accident, so that she was given an impairment rating of 5% of whole person function for the wasting alone.

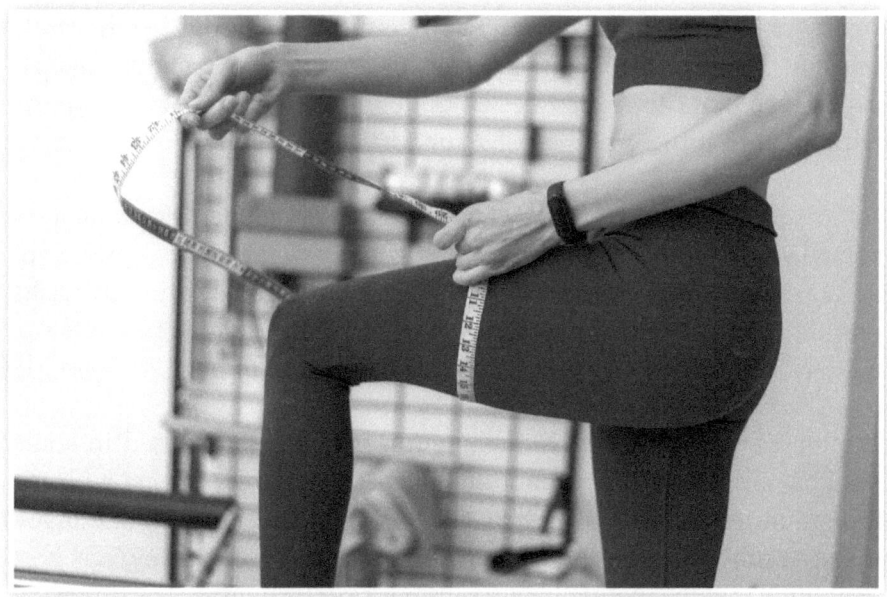

Due to some delay in bringing her case to mediation, it was necessary to re-examine her again for a contemporaneous report. In the interim, she had been examined by another medical expert who had elicited a more accurate history in which it was revealed that her muscle wasting of the thigh had predated the road traffic accident by several years. She had even been reviewed by a Neurologist, and an EMG/nerve conduction study had suggested some central cause in either the cauda equina or the spinal cord itself.

The Plaintiff's failure to mention this important point at the time of her earlier examination was a very serious oversight, and it cast doubt upon her credibility in general.

GENERAL ADVICE

What Happens To A Plaintiff During A Medicolegal Examination?

An injured claimant attends on a medical expert for an independent examination and report. The appointment will have usually been made weeks or months in advance. The party's referring lawyer is rarely present. The plaintiff is left to her or his own devices to undertake an experience that can sometimes be quite unpleasant, and some experts will not permit the presence of a support person.

As the lawyer should be aware of what is happening, solicitors sometimes, but not usually, accompany their clients. The presence of an accompanying relative or close friend is desirable. If a party asks permission to record a consultation, it should be given. In any case, modern mobile 'phones are capable of almost anything.

It is best to act as if every consultation is being scrutinised in some manner, similar to the precautions taken in treating patients with the human immunodeficiency virus (HIV), when special precautions are taken to minimise the risk of transmission. In the same way, it is best to assume that the medicolegal examiner's performance is being tested for independence.

33

LEAD ARTICLE

Who Should Be Held Liable?

It sometimes happens that more than one medical practitioner will have attended upon an injured party and the final consequences predicate the probability of negligence on the part of one and all. If there is a possibility that action against one may fail because total causation can be attributed to the other, prudence advises the claimant to sue all. The defendants are obliged to contest the issue among themselves unless it can be shown that there was no negligence at all.

An elderly lady fell, sustaining a fracture involving one hip and some associated bruising of and lacerations to her face. As well as other therapeutic measures, she underwent a total hip replacement. This is a standard approach, but, following a femoral neck fracture, there is a higher rate of post-operative dislocation. It occurred in her case. It was treated by a closed reduction, but eleven days later, the joint dislocated again. For a second time it was managed successfully with a closed reduction. The hip has remained located, though she appears to be extremely severely encumbered and ambulates little, if at all, outside the home. She sued the surgeon and the hospital staff as co- defendants.

The hospital records by way of regular written notations in the charts confirmed that the nursing staff was assiduous with warnings to her concerning post- total hip replacement precautions. Physiotherapy and occupational therapy were provided regularly and accurately to ensure that adequate training was provided, so it is difficult to see how any blame could be attributed in that direction.

In respect of the potential liability of the surgeon, the post-operative radiographs demonstrated that the implants had not been expertly positioned, that the risk of dislocation was higher than it might have been, and that he might be at least partially responsible for the unsatisfactory results.

It would be for the Court to decide on the evidence led, where, if anywhere, liability should lie. On the face of such circumstances, the paramedical staff appear to be likely to be vindicated. The surgeon is another matter.

CASE VIGNETTE

Fracture-Dislocations Of Joints Can Be Challenging

A society matron of sixty-one years of age sustained a fracture-dislocation of her dominant thumb between the first metacarpal and the proximal phalanx of the digit. Her hand had become caught in the stock she was holding when she fell whilst skiing. The applied force had bent her thumb well away from her index finger. One bone in the joint was fractured and quite markedly displaced

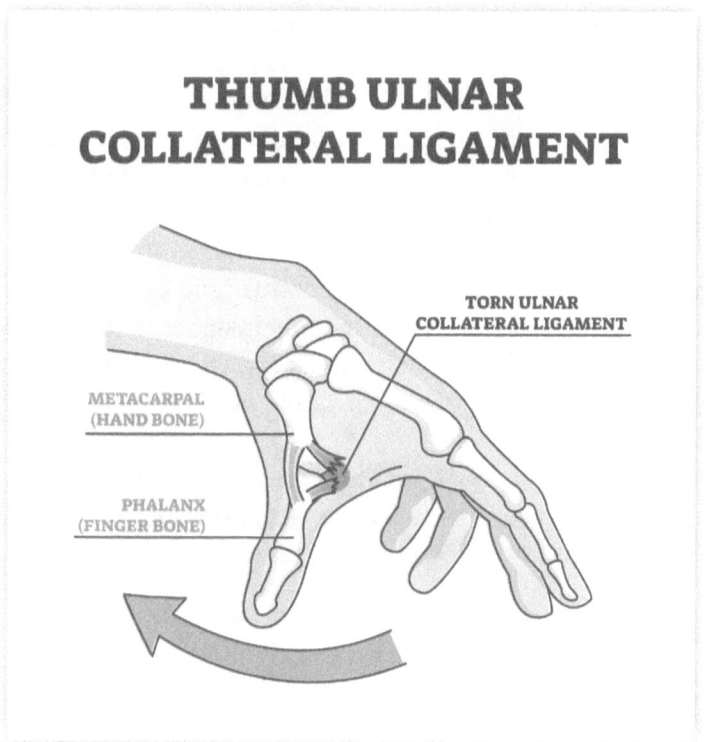

She underwent an operation which reduced and stabilised her fracture, and her thumb was held in a splint for six weeks. Though the fracture healed, an important ligament that was stabilising the joint, did not. When the splint was removed, it was apparent that the ligament was no longer functioning satisfactorily, and the thumb remained very unstable. This is sometimes referred to as "a gamekeeper's thumb". In past times, gamekeepers would snap the necks of pheasants and other game birds by holding each bird against the chest with one hand and, with the other, pushing forcibly downwards on the neck and head. The force applied to that same joint in the thumb was very similar in its mechanical nature to the force that had been applied to this lady's thumb when she fell.

She eventually underwent a second operation, with additional costs. Unfortunately, that procedure was complicated by sepsis, which necessitated further hospitalisation and intravenous antibiotic therapy. Her consequential prolonged immobility resulted in deep venous thrombi forming in one of her lower limbs, with embolisation of the clots to her lungs. As is sometimes the case, one of the emboli was of sufficient magnitude to block the bifurcation of her main pulmonary artery, resulting in sudden death. Her family experienced great anguish. What had seemed to be a simple thumb injury resulted in the loss of their wife, mother and grandmother.

A claim against the surgeon was successful. The Court held that, had the injury been treated properly in the first instance, and if the ligament had been repaired at the same time as the fracture, it was probable the unfortunate sequence of events would not have unfolded as it did.

However this may be, it is incumbent upon a treating surgeon to manage fractures and any associated dislocations totally and completely in a timely way, and not simply attend to just the fracture in isolation.

GENERAL ADVICE

Medicolegal Report Invoices - When Should They Be Paid?

There is no hard or fast rule on this matter, for commercial pressures will apply in different directions according to their circumstances. The "no-win, no-fee" adherents would probably prefer to defer payment of expert opinion invoices until final resolution of the matter. This involves an expectation that the expert should similarly carry the costs of the case, with the risk that payment may never come.

At the other end of the spectrum, the Nominal Defendant and Statutory Authorities engaged in litigation are not spending their own money, but rather that of the taxpayer, so that the time of such payment is probably of no great consequence.

Another consideration relates to a potential for resentment. Every plaintiff hopes for a supportive report on the issues of causation, liability, future economic loss and future therapeutic needs, but that is not always forthcoming. So, a plaintiff who receives an adverse report may be less inclined to pay an invoice than one who has not been disappointed.

Additionally, a reporter who seeks reassurance an invoice will be paid, might be persuaded to write a report more desirous of the payer. He may be disinclined to be distrustful of the matters expressed than might be the case if monetary conditions were removed.

It is a sensible precaution, on initially agreeing to provide an independent medicolegal opinion, to obtain a written undertaking from the requesting solicitor to be responsible for reasonable fees. The request should be accompanied by a fee schedule for relevant services including a post-file-review teleconference, the subsequent provision of a written report, if required, supply of a supplementary report if needed, and any potential court attendance(s). Payment in full before any individual service is supplied or released is advisable. The reporter can proceed, plainly not conflicted by any commercial arrangement relating to deferred payments. The opinion is not dependent upon pleasing the engaging party, and the reporter remains a free, objective advisor to the Court. Transparency about the approach adopted is of considerable merit.

Rarely does a lawyer default in payment, but if it occurs a report to the Legal Services Commission, or its equivalent, is effective.

LEAD ARTICLE

How Much Is A *pro bono* Service Worth?

It depends upon the position from which you view it. If you are the provider of a *pro bono* service, there is no direct financial gain. The recipients of such a service can benefit in that way substantially.

Some who have provided *pro bono* medicolegal services for Legal Aid plaintiffs have asked that any successful plaintiff benefiting from it would subsequently donate from their award a sum comparable to the usual fee to assist future Legal Aid services. An expectation of a positive response may be optimistic.

It's Not Just In The Medicolegal Sphere

Some practitioners also perform clinical services without a fee in suitable circumstances. Many patients are financially disadvantaged yet need prompt medical relief. Almost every medical service attracts a small fee from the Australian Government according to the Medical Benefits Schedule. It is usually only a small percentage of a proper fee, but it is something that helps to defray the costs of the practice that provides the service. The public waiting list has been excessively long, and almost punishingly so. Worthy cases should never be rejected. It is a subset of society which affords other considerable benefits to those who give.

Though the financial rewards from these services are little or none, the emotional recompense is high. The gratitude of a satisfied patient is amongst the greatest accolade any practitioner can receive. To see a disadvantaged plaintiff receive due compensation is heart-warming and nourishing.

CASE VIGNETTE

Growth Plate Injuries And Their Importance

The long bones in our skeleton grow longitudinally, with growth plates at either end of the bone, separating that part of the bone which forms a joint from that part of the bone which forms the shank. To confound those who have difficulty with spelling or pronunciation, the part that forms the joint is called an epiphysis, and the part that forms the shank is called the diaphysis. The broader segment at either end of the diaphysis is known as the metaphysis. The growth plate between the epiphysis and the metaphysis is called the physis. It is made up of cartilage cells, arranged in columns, and growing incrementally. As the basal cells mature, they form bone. They continue to grow until skeletal maturity. When longitudinal growth ceases, the entire cartilage plate ossifies (turns to bone) and the epiphysis is firmly united to the metaphysis/diaphysis. Thereafter, further growth is impossible. Prior to closure of these growth plates, young patients have an immature skeleton. In contrast adults have a mature skeleton after their physes have closed.

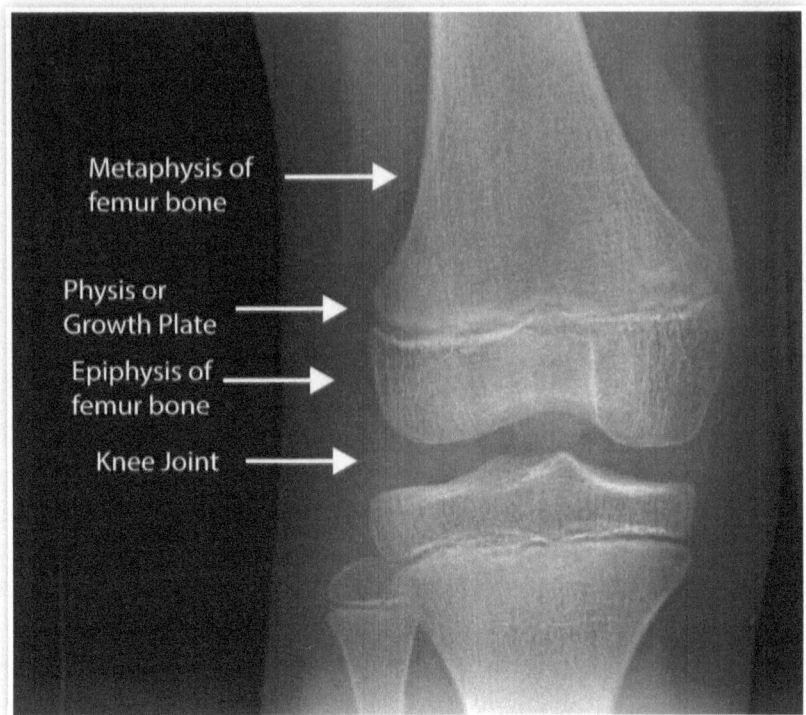

The growth plates are open. The skeleton is immature.

Fractures in long bones can occur through not only the bone (the epiphysis, the metaphysis or the diaphysis), but can also extend through the physis, the growth plate itself. These physeal injuries can be exceedingly sinister. There are five or six types, and the most used classification of them is attributed to Drs Salter and Harris from the Sick Children's Hospital in Toronto.

The importance of these fractures lies in the risk of the cartilage plate's healing prematurely, partly or wholly, with a bony or osseous bridge. If the entire physis heals with bone, longitudinal growth is lost at that level. This results in limb length inequality with shortening at that site. A clinician has several measures to manage this potential for limb length discrepancy before skeletal maturity occurs.

Another risk, probably of greater importance, is witnessed if only part of the physis heals with the bony bridge whilst the remaining part continues to grow longitudinally. This, too, will give rise to unequal longitudinal growth and an angular deformity. It can be devastating for the neighbouring joint.

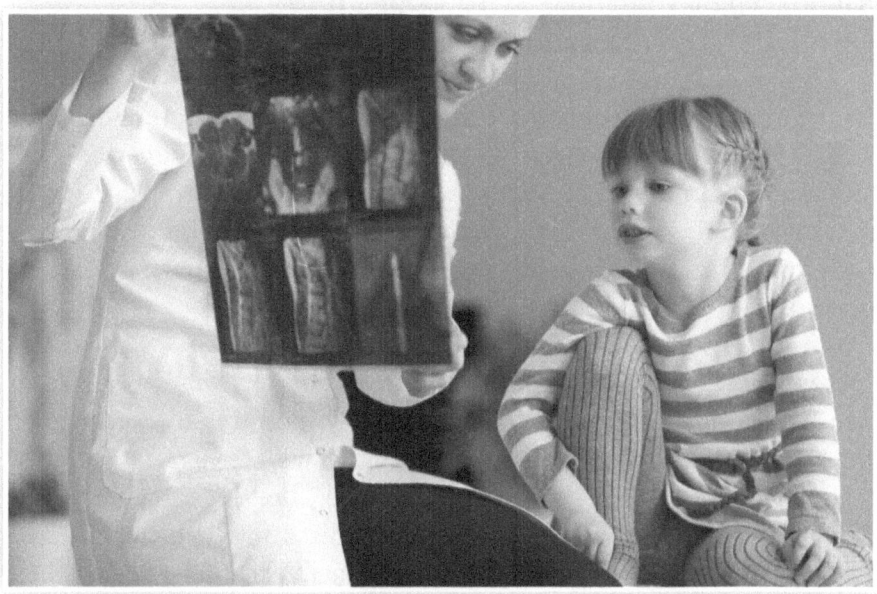

It is imperative that physeal injuries are recognised early, and managed properly by an appropriate specialist. Artificial tethering of the un-ossified side can limit or control such asymmetric growth. Alternatively, removing the post-traumatic tether may allow longitudinal growth to catch up and avoid a deformity. A Brisbane surgeon, David Vickers, was one of the early pioneers of this technique.

If a patient who has sustained an injury of this nature is a minor, it is necessary to ensure that the reporting expert is aware of these risks. What might appear to be benign and of no great significance at the time, can have much greater future significance as longitudinal growth takes place. It would produce an injustice if it had not become apparent and had not been allowed for in an award at settlement.

GENERAL ADVICE

Radiographic Imaging - Hard Copy Films Or Digital Representations?

In the radiology sphere, there has been great momentum towards storing radiographic images in a digital format. The reasons are clear. Costs can be contained, storage space is minimized, and transmissibility is vastly easier when it is through the ether. In contrast, hard copy films are expensive to produce, heavy, space-occupying, and not easy to dispose of.

Despite these respective benefits and the burdens, hard copy films still have a place. It is one that is probably more readily recognised by older practitioners, since the younger are so very attached to technical advance. All would agree, however, that it can be very time consuming to load and unload compact discs into a laptop, search through USB sticks, or otherwise search the internet for relevant files, or even compare images directly. As against that, hard copy films, properly labelled and packaged, can make all such processes very easy. Additionally, to have a hard copy on an x-ray screen in an operating theatre can be invaluable. As technology advances though, and older practitioners cease to practise, hard copy films will disappear. Not all advances are without losses. This could be one.

LEAD ARTICLE

When does 10 + 10 = 19 ?

This is a serious question, with a point to it. It has its pertinence when the American Medical Association publication, "Guides to the Evaluation of Permanent Impairment", 5th Edition (AMA 5) is used to assess impairments following functional loss. Overall, it deals with the entire body, with separate chapters dealing with the nervous system, the respiratory system, the cardiovascular system and the musculoskeletal system. There are further chapters dealing with the endocrine system, digestive system, ear nose & throat and other related structures, and more. For example, for an orthopaedic matter, it would be necessary to turn to Chapters 16, 17, 18 and sometimes Chapters 8 and 13. Chapters 16 and 17 deal with upper and lower extremity anomalies, and Chapter 18 refers to pain. Chapter 8 discusses the assessment of scarring and other cosmetic deformities, and Chapter 13 is useful for cerebral and spinal cord malfunctions.

Every Chapter contains text, figures and tables. The tables may provide guides to a medical examiner, and often include useful anatomical drawings. Importantly, they assign a percentage impairment of whole person function to a particular loss, which may be in the form of a range of motion of a joint, light touch sensation, circulation, or even part or all a limb. For example, a person who has an amputation of a lower limb through the mid-thigh suffers a loss of 36% of the whole person. One who loses a thumb is said to have lost 22% of the whole person. The rule of thumb (pun intended) requires the highest loss is combined with the next highest loss to yield a figure. That figure is then combined with the third highest loss to yield the next figure. That next figure is then combined with the fourth highest loss, and so on.

Now, let's apply the percentages prescribed by the publication to a theoretical case. A patient who has sustained multiple injuries in an exceedingly serious accident may have the following losses:

- A left sided through-thigh above knee amputation – a loss of 36% of whole person function.

- An amputation of the right thumb – a loss of 22% of whole person function.

- A serious injury to the right hip, resulting in the need for a right total hip replacement which performed to only a fair, neither good nor excellent, capacity – a loss of 20% of whole person function.

- A compression fracture in the vertebral column, resulting in a lumbosacral fusion with ongoing nerve root or radicular symptomatology, placing him in Diagnosis Related Estimate Category 5 – a loss of 25% of whole person function.

If we simply **add** 36% to 22%, to 20% and to 25%, we arrive at a total loss of 103% of the whole person. That is to say, the loss is greater than the whole! Taken even further, additional losses could be quantified for respiratory, cerebral, haemopoietic and even genitourinary losses.

The Correct Approach

In this example, the 36% loss referable to the above-knee amputation is **combined** with the 25% whole person impairment related to the lumbar spinal injury. Combined values tables are housed at the rear of the text. They yield a loss of 52% of whole person function, and not the summated 61% you might have expected.

That 52% is then combined with the 22% relating to the thumb amputation to yield a loss of 63% of whole person function.

Finally, the loss of 63% of whole person function is combined with the 20% impairment because of the poorly performing total hip replacement to yield a final impairment of 70% of whole person function. Our hypothetical individual therefore has a total impairment of 70%, rather than "103%", of whole person function.

This demonstrates a complexity of the system, which allots assessments based on single discrete impairments, without any intention that they should be treated cumulatively by simple arithmetical addition. One who uses it must then make suitable adjustments to the final calculation based on observation, experience, and common sense.

Another method rule uses a threshold of 15% of whole person function. Once it is reached, losses are combined rather than added to each other. Until that threshold, the losses are added or combined, it makes no difference. This apparent anomaly is automatically incorporated in the Combined Values Tables.

But Wait!

As with all exceptions, there are sometimes further exceptions. When adding only minor additional losses to the total, there is no difference to the result between adding and combining. For example, if a Claimant had a loss of 49% of whole person function for one part of the injuries and there was a further 1% to be added because of scarring, a total loss of 50% would be quantified by using Combined Values Tables. The additional 1% could simply have been added. Conversely, if a claimant had lost 59% of whole person function and there was a further 1% loss, the Combined Values Tables would still yield a total loss of 59%. This cross-over is at the 50% whole person impairment level.

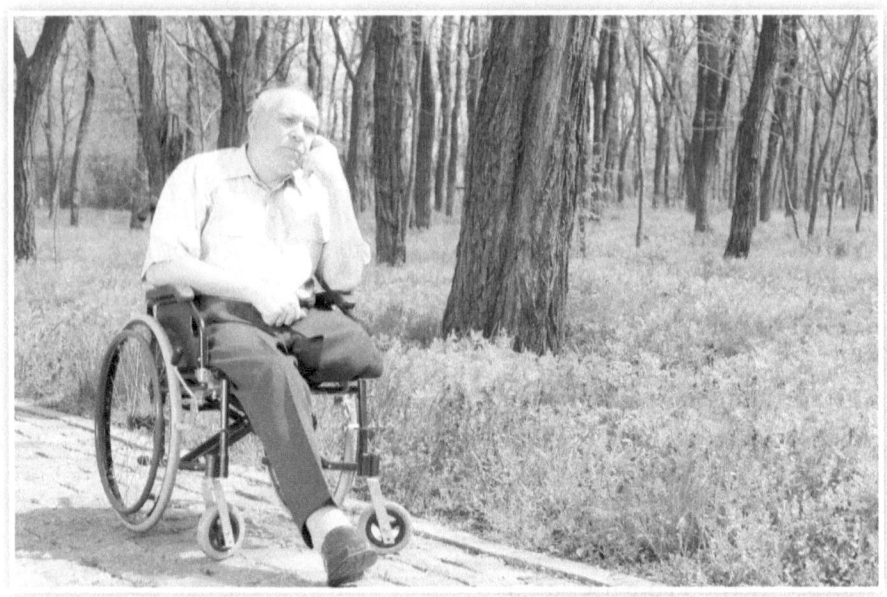

Rather than remembering these rules, simply consult the Combined Values Tables at the back of the AMA 5 Guides. They will look after you.

This explanation may be useful. Not infrequently, solicitors question the relevant arithmetic. It is based upon a misunderstanding that the respective percentages for all the losses are simply to be added rather than combined.

CASE VIGNETTE

Wrong Site Surgery

A neuroma is a swelling on a nerve. Morton first described a swelling involving the confluence of two digital nerves between two toes on the forefoot. Typically, it occurs between the third and fourth toes where the medial and lateral digital nerves coalesce. It is the mechanical theory that a slightly thickened confluence is squeezed between the metatarsal heads. As the patient ages, and the distal transverse arch in the foot drops, so do the metatarsal heads come closer together, creating a pincer effect.

A typical patient will complain of burning dysaesthesia or, sometimes, numbness on either side of the neighbouring toes. The symptoms are exacerbated by standing and walking and are sometimes best relieved by excision of the neuroma. This results in permanent numbness in that web space and on the adjacent sides of the two affected toes but relieves the unpleasant symptoms. In general terms, it is a very beneficial operation, but not always. The condition is not always between the third and fourth toes. The causal factors and their effects can appear between the first and second toes or, rarely, between the fourth and fifth toes.

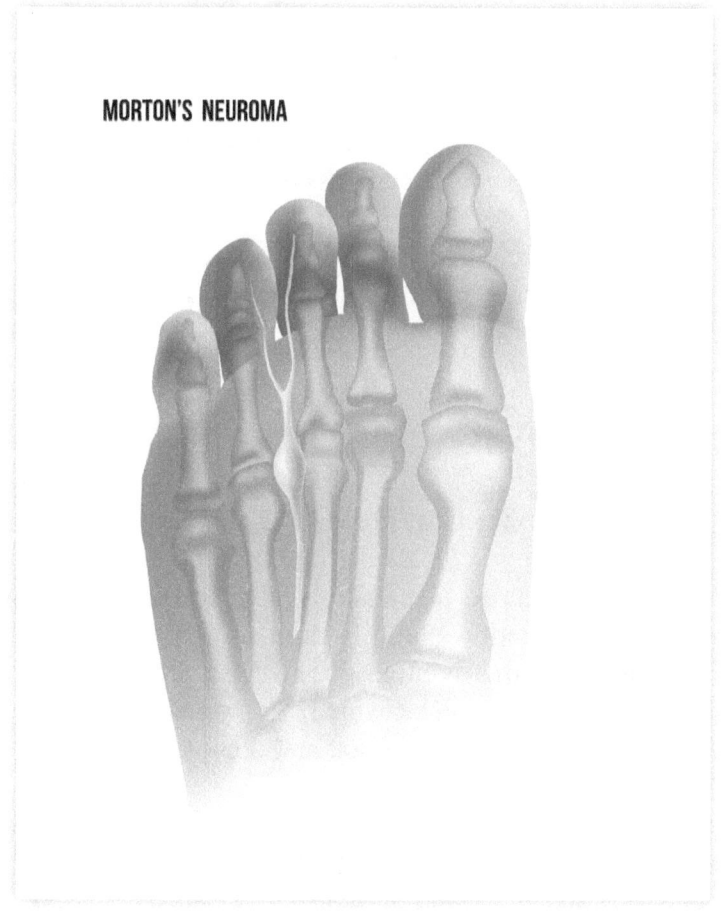

MORTON'S NEUROMA

Once, a very competent surgeon performed this operation on a patient with a Morton's neuroma. Unfortunately, he removed the nerves between two incorrect metatarsal heads, the second and third metatarsal heads, instead of the third and fourth metatarsal heads.

When the patient was no better post operatively, recognising the error, the surgeon transparently and apologetically informed the patient of the mistake and that she required a second operation. He sent her to another surgeon to perform at no expense to the patient. It was successful, and the patient was and remained asymptomatic. However, the patient was put through an additional operation with a further period of morbidity, additional expenses, and loss of earnings. The first surgeon's error was probably of a negligent nature, and a civil suit could easily have followed.

It did not follow. After non-coercive discussion, the patient elected not to sue because, she said, she still had great admiration for the surgeon, she understood that mistakes can occur, and she was also impressed by his honesty, transparency and compassion. Her benevolent employer, a friend, extended her sick leave.

This is a very valuable professional lesson. Though uncommon, mistakes of this nature do occur. "Sorry" is a very powerful word.

GENERAL ADVICE

Egos, Empires And Medical Experts

There are many facets to a medico-legal practice that bring great pleasure, both in meeting plaintiffs and in the stimulus from the intellectual challenge that is often posed. Even attendance at Court, prickly as it sometimes is, can be exhilarating, particularly if one's work has aided in the solution of a difficult and complex problem.

On another level, reading the documents accompanying a letter of instruction can be entertaining. It provides an opportunity to read the reports of colleagues and statements of the party, and to note the methods used by the former in their analyses. Some begin every paragraph with "In my opinion ...", which may be tautologous since it is understood that they are simply offering their opinions.

Others appear to be eager to put their competitors down by personally based attempts to devalue their opinions. This is contrary to their Hippocratic Oath and can be very dangerous. It can happen that the critical reporter's ego has dimmed perceptive powers so that what is reported to be an error by the colleague, was not so. The rebuff to the critic's own reputation is enhanced by the nature of the invalid criticism.

Egos, empires and medical experts are never too far apart. Witnessing their interactions can be a most interesting pastime. Professional courtesy is much more uplifting.

LEAD ARTICLE

When Experts Differ

This has been a recurring underlying theme in these discussions and deserves more focused revisitation. Differences between experts are not unusual, nor should they be unexpected. Human factors bring to an expert analysis differing life experiences and perceptions. Experts sometimes differ in their fields of study or in their education in the same field, in their own personal health spectra, in their societal attitudes, and in their degrees of sympathy or empathy. The variations can be of a multifactorial nature, and are sometimes unavoidable. They should and must be tolerated and accepted. The phrase, "agree to disagree", probably encapsulates the most reasonable approach.

There are occasions when differences are major, of pivotal importance to the outcome, and so diverse that it is likely one, or even both in some degree, is or are incorrect. This may be demonstrated by an example.

A worker in his forties had sustained a traumatic event in the region of a knee joint. He was expensively investigated pre-operatively by means of an ultrasound scan, a plane radiographic series, a CT scan and an MRI scan. The plane radiographs demonstrated that he already had osteoarthritis in the medial compartment of his injured knee. This is usually identified by the demonstration of a reduction in height of the joint space, indicating cartilage or chondral tissue loss, and the formation of marginal osteophytes or spurs.

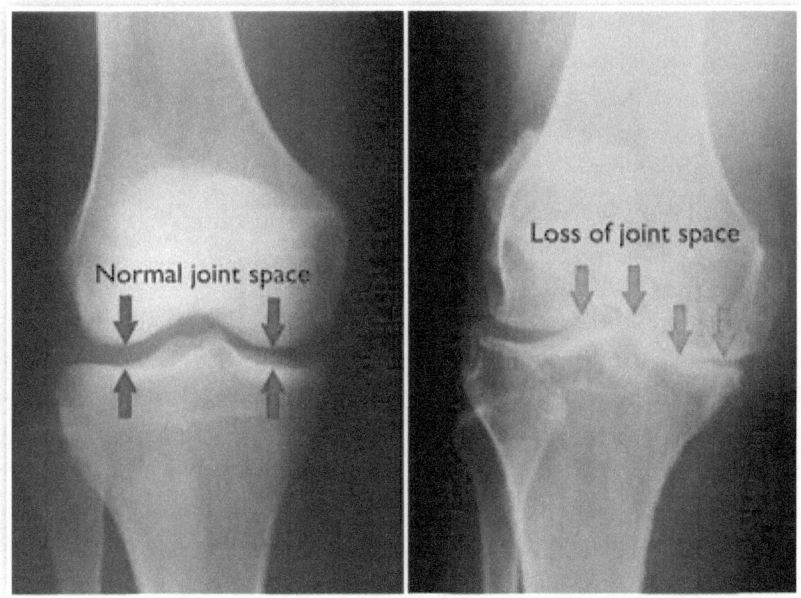

*The "joint space" is the radiolucent gap between the bones.
It is composed of cartilage.*

The MRI scan demonstrated some changes involving his medial meniscus also. It was extruded, that is, squeezed, a little outside the joint by the opposing joint surfaces, and the posterior horn was torn.

An orthopaedic surgeon performed an arthroscopic procedure. The torn cartilage, the meniscus, was trimmed, and the joint was thoroughly lavaged, that is, washed out. Not much more was done.

Unfortunately, the patient's post-operative clinical course was disappointing. His pain failed to settle, his joint was regularly swollen, he had difficulty with standing and walking, and he could not return to his pre-accident labouring work. Over the next two or three years, serial radiographs were performed and, despite his poor clinical state, the evolving radiographic changes were minimal. The measurable joint space narrowing did not progress much.

The medicolegal analysis, therefore, would result in a finding of an impairment measurement consisting predominantly of his pre-accident changes revealed on the x-rays (Table 17-31 in the AMA 5 Guides yielded 8%) and a small allocation of 1% only, according to Table 17-33, because of the partial medial meniscectomy. Thus, only one-ninth of it could be linked with the accident.

An opposing opinion from another reporter was tendered. He had viewed the same plane x-rays taken at the time of the accident and believed that the images were normal.

Importantly he opined they were completely different from those performed two or three years later. Presumably, he had viewed the MRI scan examination also. He apparently did not appreciate the joint space narrowing, or the degree of extrusion of the medial meniscus that were already present at the time of the accident. Consequently, he attributed all the changes visible at the time of his medicolegal examination to the accident, and that no apportionment was necessary. Although opinions may reasonably vary, error is also possible.

In a situation such as this, the appropriate further course for resolution lies with the requisitioning of a third opinion. A conclave of the experts may be useful too. It is best if there is agreement between the opposing parties for such a course.

If the action settles without a trial, it is desirable and a matter of courtesy for the reporters to be informed of its basis insofar as the conflicting medical issues lay apart. This is a valuable learning tool.

CASE VIGNETTE

How Valuable Are Photographs Of The Accident Site In Assessing Injuries Sustained?

Relatively useful. Extreme departures of the degree of actual injuries from those expected from the degree of damage to participating vehicles or other instruments of harm, can occur. Some passengers may escape unscathed despite their vehicle's being completely wrecked. Conversely, what might be very minor damage to a vehicle could be associated with some significant physical injury. In general terms, however, the injury spectrum and severity increase proportionately to vehicle damage.

Some years ago, a female driver's vehicle had been struck from the rear by another. The total extent of the combined damage was confined to one plastic indicator light cover. It was replaced for AUD$84.50. From this, it might have been expected that the forces applied to the female driver's car were relatively minor and unlikely to have caused her any serious injury. During her period of post-injury assessment, radiological investigations confirmed evidence of a fracture in her thoracic spine. It was assumed by the expert reporter that the fracture was caused by the accident. Importantly, the reporter did not enquire about previous thoracic injuries, and the claimant was silent on the issue of an equestrian accident as a teenager. Equally surprisingly, the insurer's expert remained ignorant on the matter too.

The claimant's solicitor engaged in correspondence with the offending driver's insurer. A considerable sum was requested by way of settlement. It was a clerk in the insurer's office, holding photographs of the minimal damage sustained, who was less certain about causation. She repeated a search of medical records. The initial review had been cursory at best. As the investigation was reopened and evolved, the truth was discovered. Each party bore its own costs and the matter settled.

This shows that, although it is not necessarily accurately predictive of injury severity, the extent of relevant vehicle damage can play some part in the final analysis.

GENERAL ADVICE

Are MRI Scan Examinations Overused?

Yes!

MRI scan examinations are expensive, useful predominantly for soft tissue injuries, and should be employed only as an adjunct to a thorough clinical examination.

Until a few years ago, only specialists could order MRI scan examinations. That privilege has since been extended to general practitioners, who can now order MRI scan examinations for some anatomical regions, and the number of those regions has increased. For example, if, as is common, a patient presents to a general practitioner with some form of knee pain, rather than taking a full history, performing a thorough examination, and attempting to make an accurate clinical diagnosis, the practitioner will refer the patient immediately for an expensive MRI scan. Often, relatively minor changes, not requiring any significant therapeutic intervention, are noted, and are commonly of a variety that would settle on their own accord. This expense was needless and should not have been incurred.

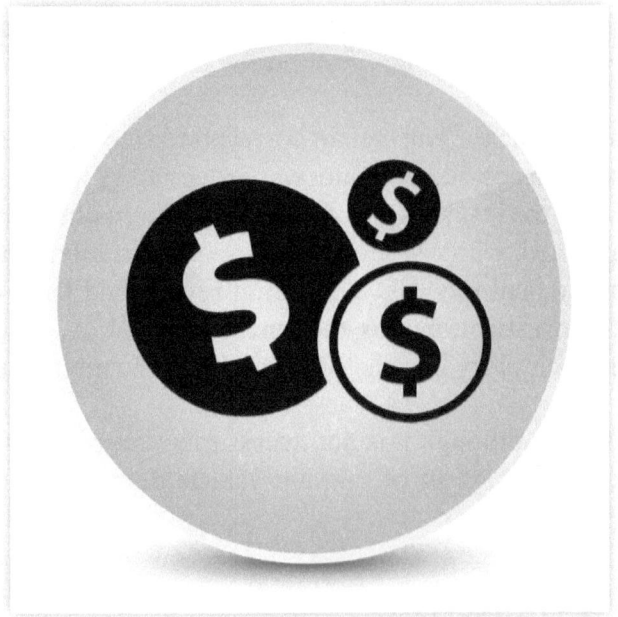

Further, MRI scans of the lumbar spine invariably show some "abnormality", even in teenagers. The aberrant findings are usually asymptomatic, and of no clinical significance. Despite that, some radiologists "over report" the significance of such findings, perhaps to justify the expense. In litigation, excessive importance can be attributed to these normal variations. These matters should be exposed. Like all investigations, MRI scan examinations should be reserved for those cases where the differential diagnosis cannot be distilled to a primary cause.

LEAD ARTICLE

Conduct Money - How Far Will 30 Bucks Stretch?

Since "subpoena" literally means under punishment, which would happen to one who disobeys it, a subpoena can be an efficient way of ensuring that a witness will attend Court when required. Typically, it is served only on those of whose attendance the party to the action requires but is not assured of. Most witnesses can be expected to attend voluntarily. So is it with an expert witness engaged by a party. A subpoena is usually not required, particularly because of a positive relationship between the medical and legal professions. The concept is to have medical experts attend between clinical commitments and interposing them in the trial as soon as reasonably possible. This sometimes extends to the point of having a witness, who is while giving evidence, stand down until the expert has been heard.

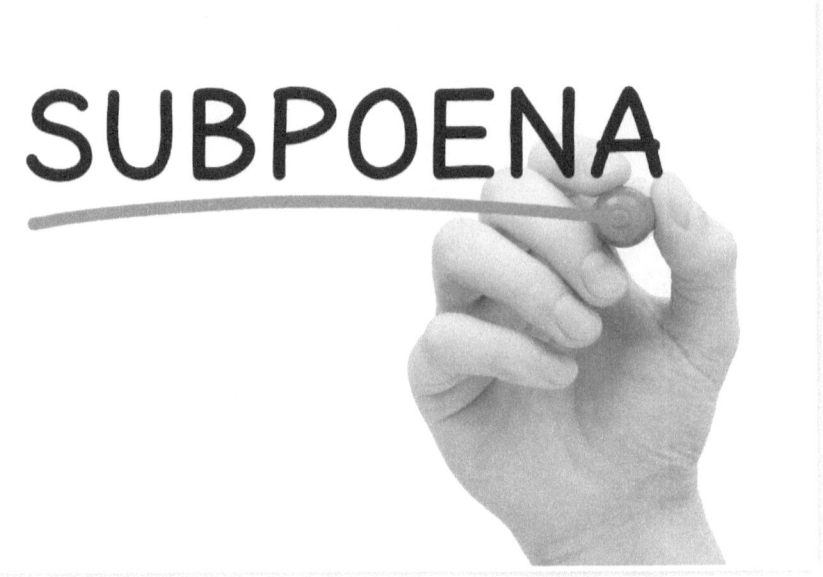

Occasionally, experts receive subpoenas, accompanied by conduct money which can be grossly inadequate. For example, if a city medical specialist was subpoenaed to attend a Court in a rural town on a specified morning at 10:00am, and thereafter until called to give evidence at a three-day hearing, conduct money of the order of AUD$30 would certainly not be recompense for the costs of travel and accommodation. The loss of earnings would far exceed standard witness' fees. On one such occasion, a medical expert refused to answer the subpoena unless given an undertaking by the solicitor who had issued it to be responsible for reasonable fees. It was not given, and the solicitor was reported to the Legal Services Commission.

Court appearances should be arranged by mutual consent, with proper allowances for expenses and fees. Disruptions should be, and usually are, minimised by co-operation on both sides of the record in the action before the Court.

CASE VIGNETTE

Bad Luck Or Negligence?

A seventy-three year old immigrant had been quite active, playing tennis, walking regularly and riding a bicycle daily. He injured his right hip joint whilst playing tennis a few weeks prior to his first presentation to his local medical officer. The doctor was perplexed but planned for an MRI scan examination and referred him to an orthopaedic surgeon.

The surgeon identified degenerative changes on the MRI scan but considered that a non- operative approach would be appropriate. The patient re-presented six months later and, according to his account, his pain was much the same. The surgeon recommended a total hip replacement. The patient claimed that he trusted the doctor implicitly, and it was for that reason that he proceeded. Unfortunately, some technical errors occurred during the hip replacement and in addition, he had a later septic complication.

An expert's advice was sought on two factors that were in issue. The first was whether the hip replacement was indicated, which is a difficult circumstance to assess in hindsight, and best judged by those present at the time. It is noteworthy that the orthopaedic surgeon had seen him on two occasions, six months apart, and on the first occasion, recommended a non-operative approach. The plane radiographs and the MRI scan examination demonstrated quite severe disease and the patient was in his seventies. On balance, it is more probable than not that the recommendation to proceed towards a hip replacement was reasonable.

The second issue related to the technical errors that occurred during the hip replacement, and particularly, whether they were related to the subsequent sepsis. There was no such link. Septic complications occur in just under 1% of hip replacements and, despite the best of endeavours, there is little more that can be done The notations showed that it was apparent that the surgeon had taken every recognised precaution to prevent a septic outcome.

Further, the technical errors were relatively minor. The test to be applied is whether the performance on the part of the surgeon was equivalent to, or better than, what would be expected of an average orthopaedic surgeon in Australia at the time. Alternatively, was the surgical performance equivalent to that of a reasonable number of his peers. Again, on the balance of probabilities, his performance was not legally negligent.

Ultimately, this has been a very unfortunate outcome for the patient. He is now far worse off than he had been and, in retrospect, would have been better off by avoiding surgical intervention. As the saying goes, "Hindsight is better than foresight by a damned sight".

GENERAL ADVICE

Medical Negligence Assessments

Litigants are becoming increasingly aware of the existence of medical negligence, and its potential for appropriate compensation. Orthopaedic surgeons are not exempt, and negligent acts do occur among them. Previous chapters have dealt with the difference between complications and negligence. That is not part of this discussion. Instead, it is directed at this increasingly important feature in medicolegal reporting. Frequent and close dialogue between the legal and medical professions is to be recommended. It is not intended to deter or dissuade litigants, but rather to ensure that investigation towards possible litigation is taken in the right direction, particularly in the area of orthopaedic advice. Much time, energy and money can be saved, and anguish avoided, by early file reviews and informal conversations between legal advocates and the orthopaedic advisor.

Can This Turn Sour?

A common scenario involves the case of a patient who has experienced a suboptimal outcome, following a joint replacement procedure. The early post-operative phase is notable for a lack of prior experience on the patient's part, not knowing what to expect and when to expect it. Reassurances offered by the medical attendants will serve to give some solace. As the months and years pass, and despite the absence of any identifiable cause, if unwanted symptoms persist, the patient may seek a second opinion. It is usually helpful, since, if it agrees with the first, the patient's concerns are usually allayed. If there is disagreement, one may be incorrect, and a third opinion may be indicated. Sometimes, personal factors may intervene to provoke the disagreement, but mostly, the second opinion may lead to the avoidance of serious medical intervention which has not been necessary, or desirable.

Unfortunately, the second surgeon sometimes sees himself as the "knight on the white horse" and incorrectly advises the patient to undergo revision surgery. This can be a serous error and may make matters much worse.

If there is an undeserved adverse outcome, the patient is rightly angry and aggrieved, but the negative emotions may be incorrectly directed at the first surgeon if the second surgeon is the culprit.

In these circumstances, it is advisable, at an early stage, to ask a reliable expert for a dispassionate opinion, which should lead to a review of the literature and a list of the correct questions to be asking before the matter is proceeded with. An expert from an outside jurisdiction may minimise the risk of interpersonal conflict.

38

LEAD ARTICLE

Reputation

It may be a professional practitioner's most important asset. The word, "reputation", is frequently used in assessing a person's performance, personality or integrity. It can be defined as:

The beliefs or opinions that are generally held about someone or something

… or …

A widespread belief that someone or something has a particular characteristic.

Several side issues emerge from these:

1. The words, "generally" and "widespread", indicate that the views of more than one, or two or even a few persons are necessary. Those of small groups or cliques are insufficient. The accuracy of the reputation ascribed is directly proportional to the size of the corpus of opinion.
2. "Beliefs" or "opinions" can be based on fact or hearsay. Facts are best served by personal experience, though even this test can be unreliable. The experience of the opinion holder may be flavoured by bias, misconceptions and subjectivity.

These negative factors may be present, but unrecognised. Assumed facts may be based upon inaccurate interpretations of observations. Unless the person whose reputation is under scrutiny is given an opportunity to explain, an erroneous impression may be retained. Inquisitive dialogue can help to avoid this.

Hearsay is infected with a further factor endangering acceptance. It relies upon the reliability and freedom from any credibility disqualifications of a person other that the one who attests the answer to the question. It is akin to rumour, so a reputation should not be constructed on it. There are several further reasons, such as the presence of laziness, a perceived lack of importance and general disinterest. More malignant reasons include jealousy, insecurity, vindictiveness and vengefulness on the part of the purveyor of the disinformation or of its ready receiver. The greater the number of steps from the source, the higher the chance of error.

3. Does it matter? It depends on several factors. Variables will include the seriousness of the matter, the depth of any inaccuracy, the adverse effect it might have on the maligned party, and the magnitude of is reach.

Reputational Damage

Sometimes a poor reputation is deserved, the disparagement will be accurate, and the subject will be obliged to accommodate its consequence. But if it is unreasonable, unfair and sprung from purely negative emotions of uncertain validity, it is not justified, and well-deserved respect is denied. Its downstream effect on others is also unjustified.

The solution for the victim is not easy to determine. There are several candidates. "Time is the great healer", "Don't get mad, get even", "Karma – what goes round comes round". None is satisfactory. Instead, leading by example, focusing on the good, maintaining perspective, and just getting on with the short lives we all have is probably the wisest combination.

All this has relevance for medicolegal reporters, their opinions, and their deftness in handling the opposing opinions by others. It is healthy to have debate. The presence of opposing views sometimes means that one is incorrect. Being right in the end is better than remaining wrong, and a capacity to change an opinion when one should is a desirable trait. A remaining rational difference of opinion can be accommodated with respectful acknowledgement of confluent assessments, and an exposé of any differences that might exist. In this it is essential that the holders of competing views remain focused on the merits of the matter, and not on the person who opposes.

CASE VIGNETTE

The Erosive Effects Of Time

A report was requested on the injuries of a person who had sustained a significant lumbar spinal injury well over a decade before. Eight years before the request, he had an operative discectomy that was apparently quite successful. Three years later, he presented with an epidural abscess. Complications of this nature are exceedingly rare. Sepsis following an operative procedure on the lumbar spine is usually apparent within days, weeks, or possibly even months. A hiatus of three years is very unusual. An unprovoked or *de novo* septic event occurring in the lumbar spine is even more unusual.

Although the temporal link between his index surgery and the subsequent appearance of the abscess is weak, it is infinitely stronger than the abscess' occurring without any relationship at all to the discectomy. At first sight, it appeared that his claim was quite straightforward and reasonable

Difficulty arose with the original cause of his decade-old lumbar spinal problem and the need for the discectomy several years later. There was no documentary evidence other than general practitioner notations confirming that "injuries" had occurred, but none had specifically mentioned an injury to the lumbar spine itself. From a clinical perspective, it is usually possible to differentiate between a single specific incident and an injury occurring over a protracted period, such as through the repetitive application of excessive stresses and strains.

In this case, although the surgical intervention was necessary, and it probably was the focus for the subsequently diagnosed infection, the task of linking the need for the operation to the "injury" occurring well over a decade ago proved impossible.

His claim in the Court was unsuccessful.

GENERAL ADVICE

Do Injuries "Occur Over A Period Of Time"?

Yes and no!

Injuries occurring "over a period of time" are not of a single type, variety or format. Some injuries are at the minor end of the scale, and complete healing can occur during the period of insult application, or even after cessation of application of the insults. Other insults are of such great magnitude that even one application would be sufficient to give rise to some form of permanent impairment or disability.

Repetitive strain injuries, or so-called "RSI", were very common thirty years ago. Many scribes, typists and factory workers claimed to suffer from RSI around the wrist or the hand. Many millions of dollars were probably paid out on this alleged condition until the professions finally called a halt.

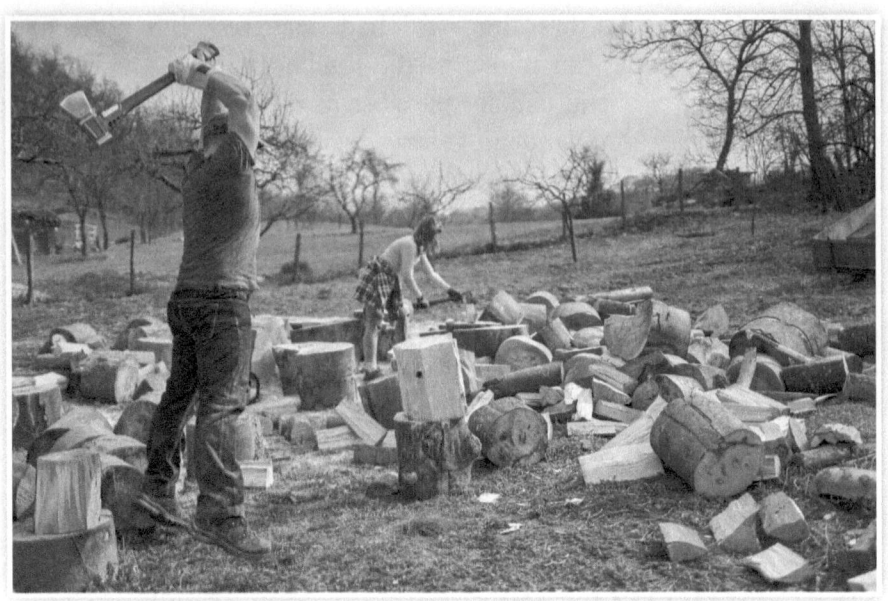

It should also be appreciated that such claimants do not engage in only remunerative activities that could give rise to injuries "over a period of time". They are also concomitantly leading a normal life. Social, recreational and domestic insults may be adding to the injury spectrum. Processing all these components and apportioning blame fairly can be almost impossible. This is not to suggest that it should not be tried, nor that the concept is unreal, but rather that the difficulties should be acknowledged. It is always much easier to deal with the analysis of the aftermath of a single serious injury.

LEAD ARTICLE

New Concepts In The Medicolegal Business Arena

For the last half century or more, we have seen sole operators acting as experts, producing reports, and defending their positions in the personal injury and medical negligence jurisdictions.

The Independent Expert

For respect, a sole operator is reliant upon reputation for quality, objectivity and transparency. Some became known as "doves", "soft touches" or "bleeding hearts", and accordingly, were favoured especially by the plaintiffs' lawyers. Others were at the much stricter end of the spectrum and were referred to as "hawks" or "sharks". Inevitably, the conflict between these reporting styles would result in actions that could be concluded only in the Court, or by both sides' agreeing to accept the opinion of a third, non-polarised expert. This situation continues, although is less common and continues to diminish.

Brokers As Partners

Over the last fifteen or twenty years, broking firms have entered the business. They corner the work from law firms that require expert evidence for their clients' affairs, have a stable of reporters covering all or most specialties and profit share with the reporter. Their share varies according to the services that they provide. For example, some will arrange for all the secretarial and reception needs, provide the professional rooms, undertake the transcription and typing, and produce the final report. The expert's only participation is to examine the plaintiff and dictate the report. The share varies from firm to firm, but generally the broker takes about 60% and the expert receives about 40% of the fee that is ultimately invoiced. This arrangement has proved to be exceedingly lucrative for the broking firms. They continue to increase in numbers, and several have sold their businesses to larger corporate entities or private investors.

Brokers As Intermediaries

More recently, a variation has been emerging. It involves a company's acting as a purveyor of medicolegal work. It solicits work from the legal profession, advertises on a website and social media platforms, and engages in personal visits. Referrals received are sent to an expert who manages the entire process through to completion without further assistance. Rather than using a profit share arrangement, it takes a booking fee (say of AUD$25) and, in addition, a percentage of the sum finally invoiced (say 5%). The fairness, for an expert, of this arrangement will depend upon one's own personal perspective. For some, it will be a very convenient model to continue to use in practicing into their twilight years. For others who lack the necessary infrastructure, the minimal assistance provided will be insufficient. They will probably continue to use the broker.

Ultimately, the way a report is solicited is irrelevant. It is the quality of the final report that should be the principal focus.

CASE VIGNETTE

What Lies Ahead?

A year 12 high school student, involved in a motorcycle accident, sustained fractures involving his tibia and fibula, distal femur and pelvis. His convalescence was complicated by a pulmonary thromboembolic event. He commenced a third-party personal injury claim, and two expert surgeons provided reports for the Court. Both accurately identified the problems that had been sustained at the time of the accident, but neither referred to long-term effects that he would experience five or more decades later.

The injuries plateaued, stabilised for a decade or so, and then began an inexorable deterioration. He has had further pulmonary thromboembolic complications, probably causally linked to a spinal fusion. He required two major joint replacements and an ankle arthrodesis. These sequelae were foreseeable.

Neither expert referred to the likelihood of these future complications. The Court was not advised of the potential, nor its probability. The award made no allowance for these eventualities.

He is in his seventies now and continues to suffer the sequelae. Retrospective compensation doesn't exist. It was an opportunity lost through ignorance.

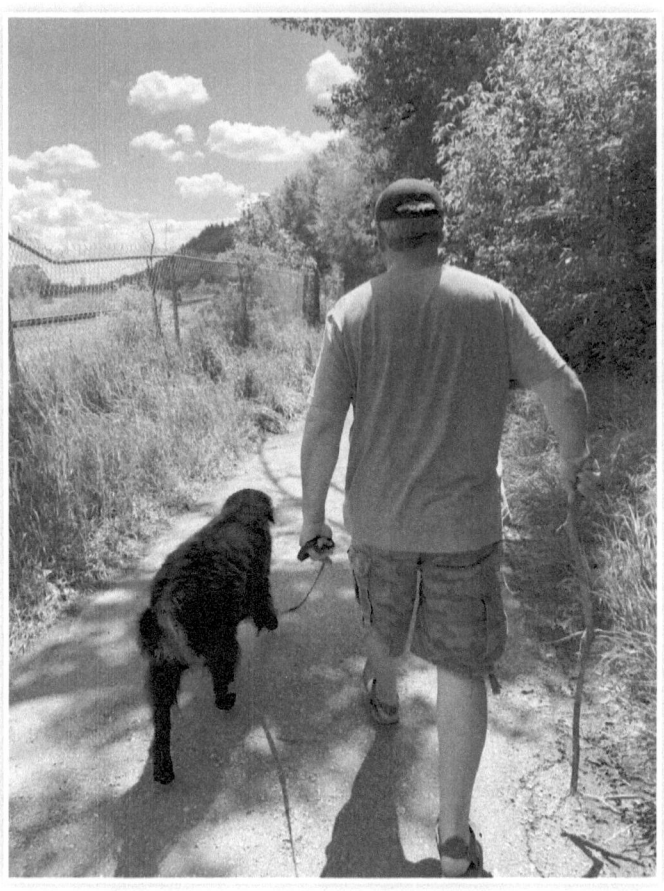

This shows that when a medical expert reports on a client, she or he should ensure consideration of any long-term adverse effects that may accrue, and the solicitors should check that it has been done.

GENERAL ADVICE

Is It Worth The Effort?

Some aggrieved patients are keen to pursue a perceived under-performing doctor for damages after an adverse result. Anger, frustration and disenchantment all fuel that desire for compensation as a recognition of the wrong believed to have been done. Some, lacking the financial backing to do so, rely upon legal firms who are prepared to take a "no-win, no-fee" engagement. These organisations must be extremely cautious. They could outlay many thousands of dollars on a fruitless search before the realities of the chances of success become apparent. Such a potentially wasteful process could be short-circuited easily by an early "off the record" chat with a medical expert in the field that may give a good indication of the likelihood of success or otherwise.

I do it frequently.

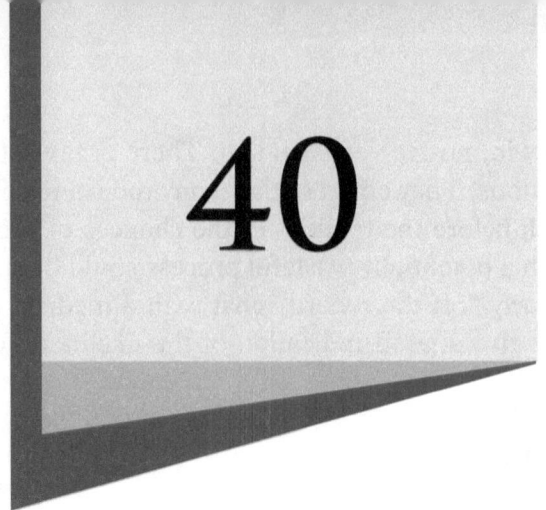

40

LEAD ARTICLE

Two In One Week---

Two medical negligence cases running in the one week were strikingly similar, despite being from different states, involving patients of different gender, and regarding different parts of the anatomy.

The first was brought by an elderly lady who had undergone a hip replacement in a southern state three years before. It appeared that the surgery was performed competently and that the post-operative course, although not as smooth as might have been hoped for, was well within usual parameters. She still suffered some ongoing discomfort.

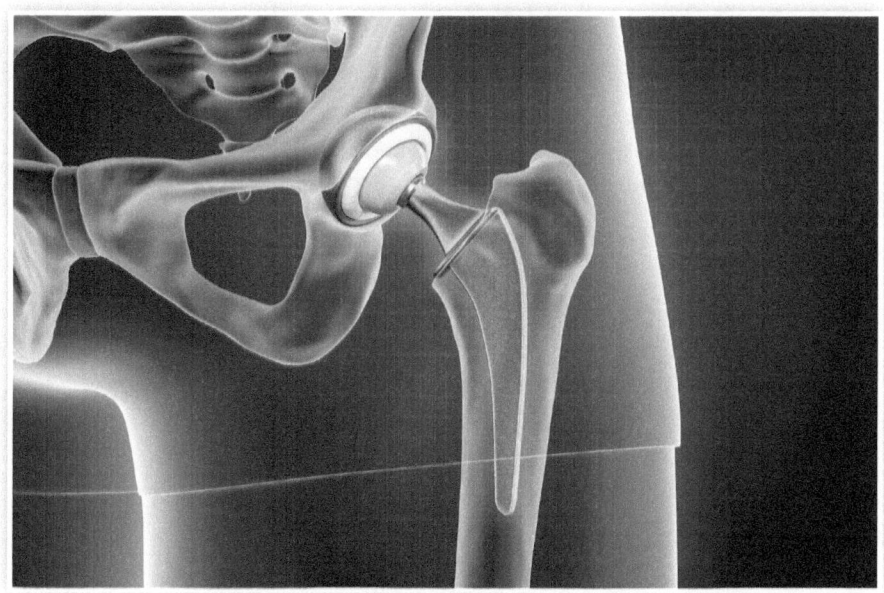

Her difficulty began when her general practitioner referred her to a second orthopaedic surgeon for another opinion. That second surgeon had a significant dislike for the first, and claimed to identify problems that, as it turned out, did not exist. He also undertook revision surgery to correct the suggested anomalies but, as there were none, understandably, it failed. The patient's anger with her condition, fuelled by comments of the second surgeon, had her intent on suing the first surgeon but, fortuitously, well-phrased comments in his report to her solicitors assuaged her discontent. He really had no case to answer. The situation of the second surgeon may well have been a different matter!

The second case involved an elderly male who had undergone a knee replacement. His surgeon had made a per-operative error and on his referral to a second surgeon, corrective surgery was undertaken. Unfortunately, during the second surgery, that surgeon also made a serious error, requiring the patient's referral to a third surgeon for yet another operative procedure. The patient sued the first surgeon, alleging that all the adverse events that followed the first surgery were due to his malpractice. Clearly, that was not the case, for the second surgeon had contributed to the need for the third surgery and the ultimate outcome.

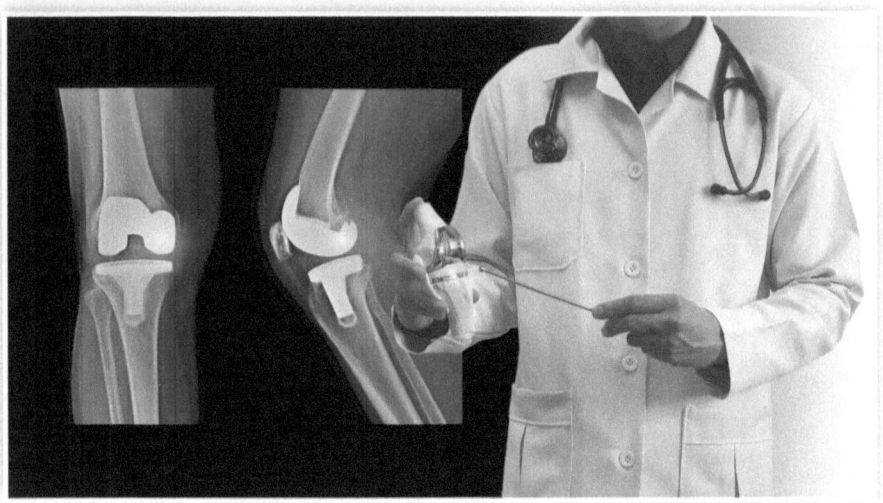

It is sometimes surprising how these events cascade into a dizzy downwards spiral. The first case was precipitated by unforgivable unworthy emotion. In the second case, there was no malign intent nor avarice. Unfortunately, the former has become a common theme.

CASE VIGNETTE

Horses Are Heavy

A twenty-eight year old secretary was visiting a local winery on a Sunday afternoon. By all accounts, she enjoyed herself enormously. The food was excellent, the wine flowed copiously, and although she was able to walk to her car, she needed considerable aid. En route to the car park, she took a detour. She had spied three horses in a nearby paddock and, because of both the influence of liquor and her love for animals, her approach to them was too close. The nearside front hoof of one trod quite excitedly on her sandalled toes.

Her state of inebriation was such that she probably did not register much feeling, though three of her digits were immediately amputated and the remaining two were quite dusky. Over the next several weeks, one of the remaining toes required amputation but the fifth digit, her hallux or great toe, was saved. Many months of rehabilitation followed.

She brought an action for damages against the proprietor of the premises, and her claim included post-traumatic stress disorder (PTSD). Although there had been no padlock on the gate to the horses' paddock, it was firmly closed and required two hands to disengage the catch. There was also a small sign, warning guests not to enter the paddock, and indicating that it was both private property and a place of danger.

Not surprisingly, her claim was unsuccessful. It was a salutary warning against long lunches.

GENERAL ADVICE

Can The Legal System Be Trusted?

Most lawyers would say "yes". They have been schooled in the system, and have considerable experience, but they belong to the club and have a vested interest. Like the members of any other profession, they are subject to influences from those sources. That is not to say that there are not strong members of goodwill who see the defects and move to repair them. They look inwards and publish their views within their profession, but do not trouble their medical colleagues with such non-medical matters, just as the national medical associations do not usually consult the law societies.

Doctors, not uncommonly, have a different view of the legal system, while they enjoy the same features in their own, albeit in different forms. Naturally, there are differences between those professions. The legal profession does not condone untruths but there have been situations where inconvenient truths are ignored. This sometimes arises because Counsel for a party must efficiently present a client's case as instructed and without rejection of those instructions. As an aside, some "unlikely instructions" have proved by the complete evidence to have been correct. Anecdotal cases of professional wrong are, just as in the medical profession, not indicative of a general state.

Honourable clinicians are not inclined to bias or dishonesty. They generally rely upon absolute and complete truth. It assists in the diagnostic process, improves the formulation of therapeutic regimens, and adheres to their Hippocratic oath. Even then, they, like lawyers, can be in genuine error.

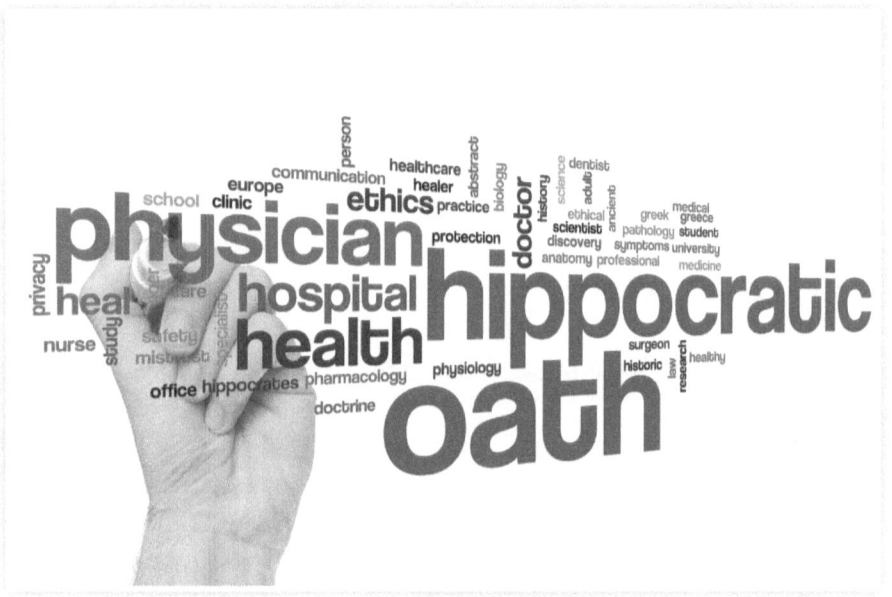

Some plaintiffs who have been through litigation appear to be dissatisfied with the system. That could well be through their own inadequacy in understanding or knowledge of all the facts, as well as their own emotional forces. They may not complain about the quantum of their award, but of what they perceive as unfairness in the whole system. They refer to the lengthy nature of the process, the large costs involved, and the unpredictability of the result.

These sometimes reflect a misunderstanding of the difficulties of the Law to provide quality justice. Obstacles provided by possible cunning and guile require disputing parties to have the opportunity to know the case they must answer and to prepare their presentation carefully.

This includes the gathering of evidence and advice as to further action, and to test the opposing case. It usually requires considerable and necessarily sequential action. Issues are referred to expensive experts, such as Counsel and medical experts, whose fees reflect the degree of their ability. In part, the process predicates the result.

Uncertainty of the result is caused by many factors, including the quality of the party's evidence, and that of his witnesses, and even if it is right, the quality of its presentation in the witness box. In the end, experienced judges can usually find their way through the difficulties set up by the parties and their witnesses, but of course, it is not always possible.

There is constant activity for Law Reform to meet such difficulties as may be met. The vagaries of human nature as revealed by the witnesses, and even in the personality of some judges, render finding any fully effective solution for this issue unlikely.

41

LEAD ARTICLE

Same Injury - Two Outcomes

Consider two twenty year old men who, on the same day, were involved in identical accidents, each injuring his left knee.

John, a third-year electrical engineering student, sustained a displaced fracture of the lateral tibial plateau within his right knee joint. The displacement was not severe, and his orthopaedic surgeon considered that it could be managed non-operatively. His limb was braced for eight weeks, and he then received some physiotherapy for two or three months.

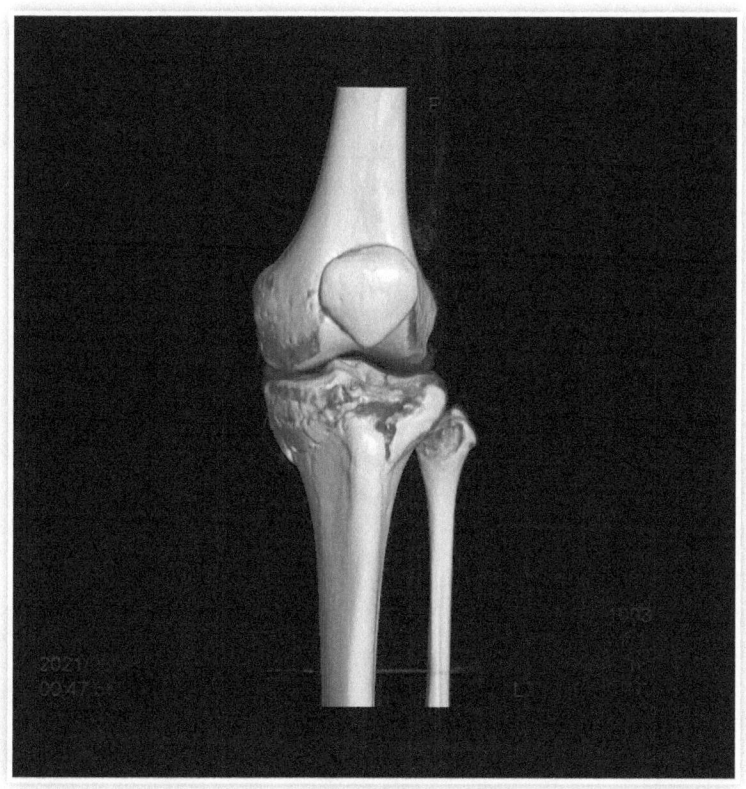

The fracture healed, and although the subsequent radiographic images confirmed that the joint was not pristine, he was able to cope with his duties as an engineer over the next few years. He avoided running and jumping, engaged in swimming and bike riding only, and his prognosis appeared to be relatively good. Clearly, he had sixty years or more of useful life ahead of him and, therefore, there was a small risk that he may develop osteoarthritis in that compartment of the joint, necessitating a total joint replacement. It is impossible to be certain as to the magnitude of the risk, but it was probably of the order of only 10% to 15%.

Peter, a marine boilermaker who had just finished his apprenticeship, had secured a job on a tugboat operating off the coast of Western Australia. It was a particularly impressive vessel and operated in tandem with another vessel in manoeuvering very large ships that were taking iron ore to Asian markets. As part of his duties, he was obliged to ascend and descend eight flights of steel steps many times during a 12-hour shift whilst tending to the engines deep in the bowels of the vessel. He also manned winches and ropes on deck. These particularly arduous duties had a deleterious effect upon the fracture that had otherwise healed satisfactorily.

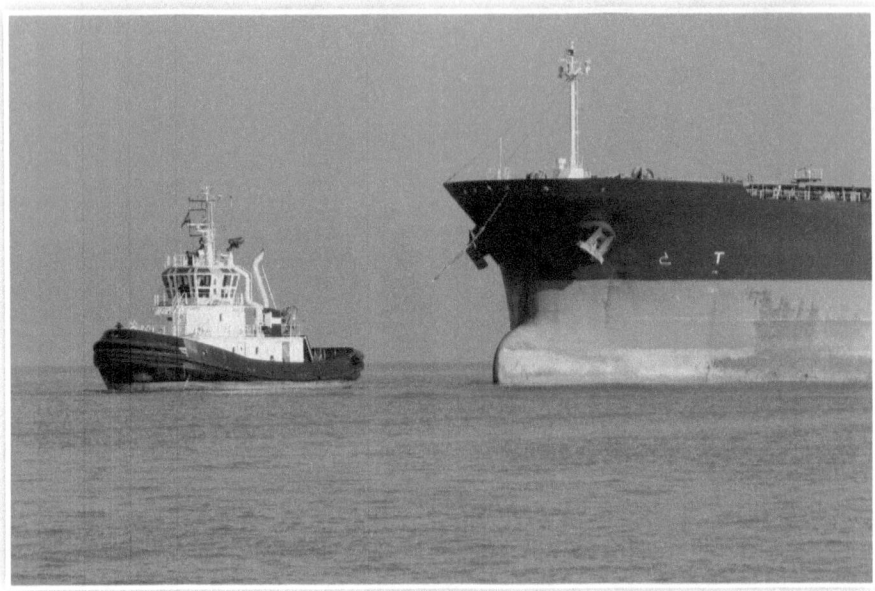

It was likely that he would develop osteoarthritis in this joint much sooner rather than later, so that he would then be unlikely to be able to continue working in this marine environment for more than the next ten or fifteen years. His chances of requiring a total knee replacement by the time he retired were probably in the order of 50% to 60%.

Because John and Peter were of the same age and had the same injury, theoretically, they would have had the same prognosis if their circumstances were similarly identical. It was the superimposition of their different work stresses that separated them so markedly. Projected lifestyles must influence civil award quanta. This is a variable, amongst many that an expert medical reporter should address. For every injury, there is a broad spectrum of possible outcomes. Every case should be assessed medicolegally upon its own merits.

CASE VIGNETTE

The Wrong Pathology

In a surgical procedure on a hip, the surgeon had completed the operation perfectly, but it was the wrong operation! He had performed an iliopsoas tendon release, believing that the patient suffered with intractable pain because of iliopsoas tendinopathy. This is a condition that usually presents with mechanical groin discomfort. The true pathology was not related to the psoas tendon, but rather to a labral tear, detachment and chondral anomaly within the hip joint itself. The iliopsoas tendon is outside the hip, while the labrum, like a cartilage in the knee, is inside the joint.

There is no real need to address the precise pathology. As it is shown in this imaginary example, attention should be focused upon doing the right thing at the right time, for the right reason on the right patient. Without this combination, adverse outcomes are likely to be witnessed.

Is It Common?

This problem strikes at the core of diagnostic acumen. All doctors are capable of errors. An incorrect diagnosis might lead to an incorrect therapeutic regimen. The patient's condition may not improve, and may be made worse.

It is difficult to know how often this occurs, but it is probably not rare. It is not enough to say, "Let's try this first. If it doesn't work, I've got another idea". This could continue for some time, with the trial of many new ideas. How much patience must the patient have?

This issue becomes very important when an erroneous diagnosis, and, consequently, the wrong treatment plan, cause serious and irreparable harm. Unless recognised early, it becomes potentially disastrous for the patient, and the first foments of a medical negligence claim.

GENERAL ADVICE

The Wrong Direction

There is a steady increase in the number of cases of alleged medical negligence, but that does not mean that there is necessarily a higher incidence of medical negligence, allowing for the increase of population. A lower threshold for litigation is another factor. There is a very important difference between a complication in the treatment of an injury, on the one hand, and the result of negligence on the part of the treating doctor. Without medical training plaintiffs often have difficulty in recognising the difference.

A claimant who had undergone an open reduction and internal fixation of a fracture around the ankle joint experienced subsequent infection that necessitated multiple further operative procedures. A very undesirable long-term destruction of the joint ensued. His solicitor had the malpractice gun pointed squarely at the surgeon.

His initial treatment, including the operative fixation of the fracture, was excellent and beyond reproach. The patient had been discharged from the care of the hospital where it had taken place and returned to another State. Ten days following the operation, he presented to a hospital in his home city with symptoms and signs consistent with an infection. That hospital took no appropriate action for six days. Eventually an Infectious Diseases Physician suggested to the Orthopaedic Department that the patient may require operative drainage and lavage of the ankle joint.

It was irreparably damaged, not by the original injury, but by the aftermath of the unrelenting sepsis that ensued. Pus is powerfully chondrolytic, that is, cartilage destroying, for which the emergency treatment is surgical drainage and, if needed, antibiotics.

Though the facts and reasons are not known, there may have been some serious under-performance by the second Orthopaedic Unit for having taken no action in respect of this pus-filled joint for 6 days. The plaintiff's original action was misdirected, and cogent advice resulted in the legal action's being more appropriately directed.

The Message?

Good orthopaedic advice, obtained early, can help differentiate between complications and negligence, and properly direct legal action, should it be required.

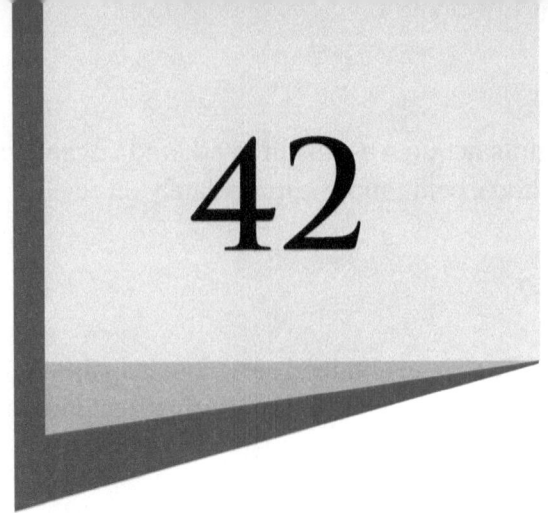

LEAD ARTICLE

Are X-rays Necessary?

It is important for legal colleagues to understand that the diagnostic and therapeutic programme adopted by medical practitioners is almost universal. The process involves the gleaning of a full history of both the relevant injury and of all relevant prior medical features, the performance of a thorough clinical examination, and then a review of appropriate ancillary investigations. More than 85% of diagnoses can be based upon the history and examination alone, but the ancillary investigations increase the diagnostic accuracy to the high 90%'s.

Of all the ancillary investigations available to orthopaedic surgeons, plane radiographs are probably the most valuable. They allow them to see, in two dimensions (and that's why they are called "plane" and not "plain"), the probable pathological processes involved. Education enables a translation between the radiographically created images, and pathological processes. Without the radiographs, the differential diagnosis list can be very long, but if appropriate investigations are available, it can be reduced to one or two probabilities only.

In the medicolegal sphere, they are often of vital importance. Negligence cases rely heavily upon images taken before, during and after an alleged negligent event. Opinions can be formulated on the likelihood of progression of the injury in the absence of the alleged negligence, the true effects of the allegedly negligent intervention, and the natural history of the aftermath.

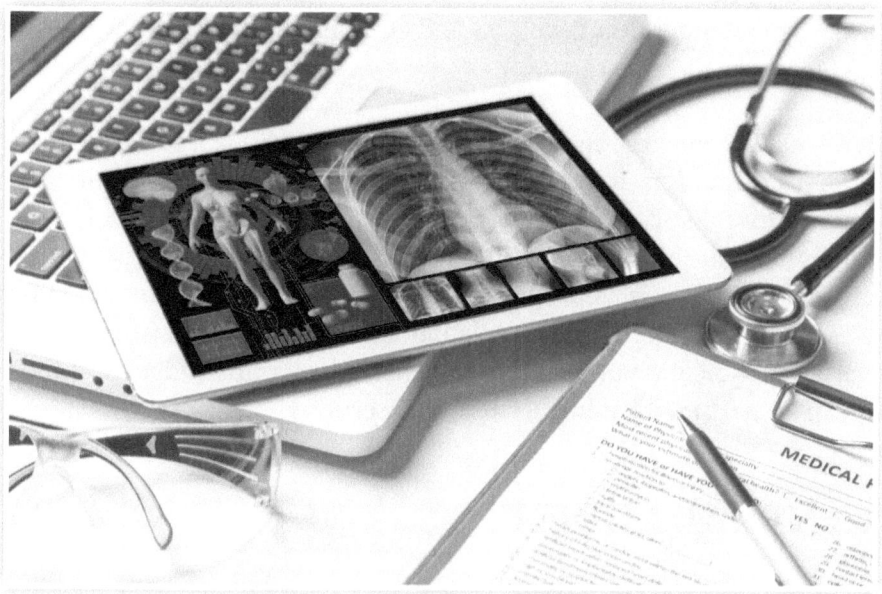

If briefs to medical experts, seeking an opinion on negligence or causation of harm, completeness is vital. All proper ancillary investigations should be included.

CASE VIGNETTE

How Hard Should One Look To Past Medical History?

A plaintiff claimed to have sustained a knee joint injury "over a period of time" of about two months. He had been engaged in arduous work practices as a railway fettler laying new tracks. Uneven terrain was common, objects requiring moving were heavy and access was often difficult. He was referred for assessment. These "over a period of time" injuries are always difficult to assess. Without a precise description of a specific event, it is difficult to link a clinical circumstance to something that is vague and most unspecific. Nevertheless, two experts attributed his current condition wholly and solely to the work practices, but, unfortunately, they had not deeply investigated the plaintiff's medical history. He had been a particularly active soccer player at a high level for many years, a triathlete of some standing, a rock climber, and an avid gym attender doing weights and circuits seven days per week. He had never been sedentary.

It is hardly surprising that he had some radiographic and MRI scan examination findings of degeneration within his joint, and it was unrealistic to believe that six or eight weeks of work were totally responsible for his condition. As a matter of common sense, apportionment was appropriate. It did not imply that the claimant was prevaricating. A simple explanation of the full circumstances and objective indications is enough to satisfy the Court. Judges live lives too. The past medical history requires scrutiny.

GENERAL ADVICE

Will Personal Injury Litigation Ever Stop?

It is something like a self-saucing pudding, never diminishing. In countries with "no fault" insurance, for example, New Zealand, it is uncommon. Whether a patient is in a hospital bed because of severe multi-trauma from a road traffic accident or because of contracted hepatitis would not matter, there would be compensation.

Under other systems, it would be necessary either to identify a culprit or, alternatively, to sue the Nominal Defendant if the culprit cannot be found or cannot be sued. Under these systems, there are fees to be won by lawyers and expert reporters, and potential benefit for the plaintiff. None of these would ordinarily be keen to end a system which, however, imposes serious cost on society.

Refinement will continue and is to be applauded. Avarice will never disappear though and the sauce for the pudding is unlikely to dry up.

LEAD ARTICLE

Shifting Sands

The rate of the progressive evolution of medicine is extraordinary, especially in trauma surgery. Whereas thirty years ago, teenagers or patients in their early twenties would spend six weeks or more in traction following a femoral shaft fracture, many are now given operative internal fixation, and are inpatients for no more than a day or two. In this way, considerable savings can be achieved in hospitalisation, which usually costs between AUD$2,000 and $2500 per day. Other real savings include reduced loss of remunerative engagement, diminishing the hidden cost of social and mental health disturbances, and general costs.

Not all advances are so meritorious. Small fortunes are made by hip and knee arthroplasty manufacturers, sponsors and distributors. Despite the excellent performance of the current bevy of hip and knee replacement devices, there is still a constant search for the "holy grail". On reviewing the Australian Orthopaedic Association National Joint Replacement Registry (AOANJRR) over the last decade, it is apparent that newer devices do not perform any better than their predecessors. Sometimes they perform worse, and invariably they cost a great deal more than their predecessors. Research is commendable. There is still room for improvements in design, and creative intent should not be thwarted, but high-level evidence should be forthcoming before superior clinical performance can be claimed for these recent innovations.

Those with most to gain are not the best arbiters. Governments, health insurers, hospitals and medical professionals have a duty to society. Expenditure is to be based on evidence. This is where the medicolegal perspective resides. The latest, greatest medical device might be implanted with alacrity for a few years into unsuspecting patients. Only then is premature failure recognised, revision surgery required, and the distasteful saga begins. History shows that blame shifting is rampant, responsibility is denied, and proof is mysteriously clouded. Beware.

CASE VIGNETTE

Osteoporosis Of Pregnancy

Osteoporosis is demineralisation of the collagen structure in bone. It can present clinically as a cause of fractures, even by minimal force, and radiographically by bones that are far less radio-dense than normal. It is often associated with age, and especially in females. It can also be associated, rarely but in a spectacular fashion, with the third trimester of pregnancy in younger women. Mothers at or about the age of thirty years appear to be particularly vulnerable and it is during the third trimester that hip pain, either unilateral or bilateral, is noted.

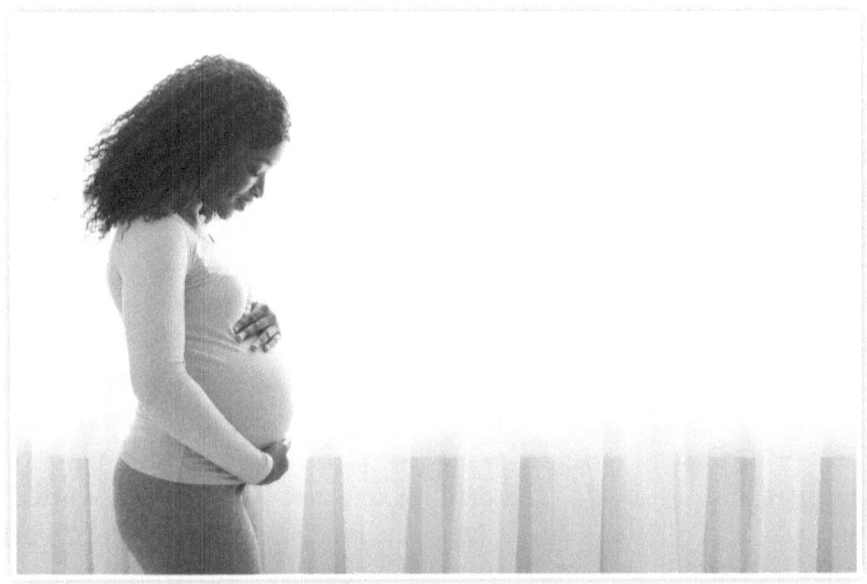

The diagnosis is initially made by the suspicious, inquiring clinician. It is best confirmed with an MRI scan examination, and treatment modalities will differ according to the extent of the lesion that is identified. Ideally it is identified in its earliest phases, before a fracture of the femoral neck occurs and before anything more than rest and observation are required. It resolves after confinement.

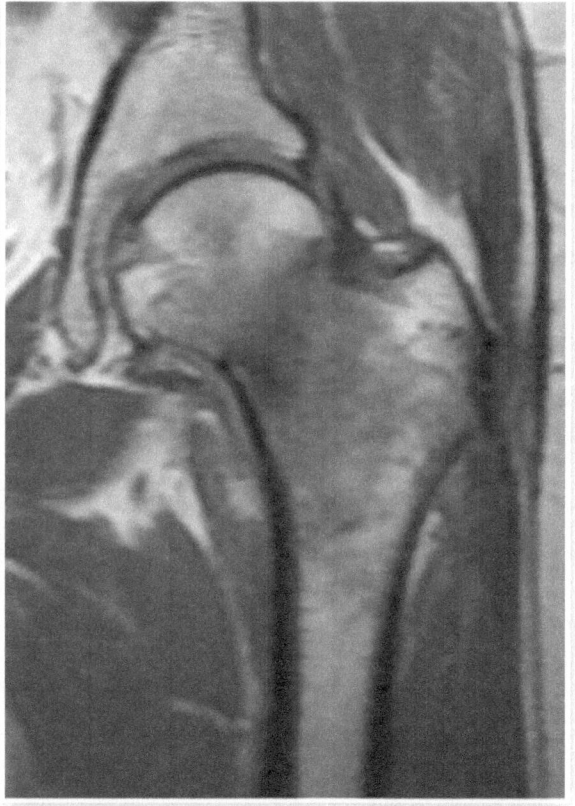

The MRI scan is a sensitive indicator of osteoporosis

Sometimes, if the diagnosis is delayed, a fracture of the femoral neck will occur. If it is incomplete or undisplaced, it can be managed relatively easily by internal fixation. This is not very difficult, subject to a caveat that anaesthesia in late pregnancy poses special challenges. Most fractures will then proceed to sound osseous union, with little or no long-term sequelae. If the diagnosis is delayed, the most undesirable sequence is that a fracture occurs, it becomes displaced, and the risk of non-union, delayed union or avascular necrosis of the femoral head increases exponentially. If the fracture is displaced, and the recognised complications ensue, a total hip replacement might be needed.

Then it becomes more complicated. The hip replacement will solve the problem initially, but it is undesirable in the case of patients in their early thirties. Hip replacements have a finite life span and, theoretically, 10% of those patients will require a revision by their early fifties. Of those, a further 20% will require a second revision in their seventies. Even a third revision may be required in the patient's eighties, which is becoming more likely, given contemporary actuarial longitudinal life studies. As the number of operations increases, so does the risk of complications, cost, and suffering.

It is important therefore that all clinicians involved in obstetric care have at least a high index of suspicion for this unusual and uncommon condition. Early diagnosis, proper orthopaedic care and judicious rehabilitation can effect an excellent outcome. Otherwise, it can be far from desirable.

GENERAL ADVICE

Patient Demeanour

All of us are subject to bias to a greater or less degree, and with a wide variety of recognition of its presence in oneself. Even the most revered judges will have some preconceptions based upon past experiences. Medical experts are no different. Steps should be taken to exclude its influence in circumstances where it might be operative. Lawyers sometimes fear that a very upright judge, before whom they are appearing and whose natural bias would favour their case, might lean over too far backwards in trying to overcome his self-perceived bias.

So it can be with plaintiffs. Patients who complain far too much and in an unpleasant way, are less likely to be taken seriously than an individual who presents in a mainstream manner. Embellishment is expected but limits exist for all of us. Very occasionally, patients at the opposite end of that spectrum present for examination. They have suffered very severe injuries, yet complaints must be dragged out of them. It is this latter group, as rare as it is, that often evokes the more sympathetic reports from even the most sceptical reporters. This should not be encouraged in patients, but embellishment should be discouraged.

44

LEAD ARTICLE

'You Can't Be Serious!'

This is a famous phrase, commonly attributed to John McEnroe. Some plaintiffs feel the same. Many have been subjected to quite significant injuries which have had major life-altering effects, sometimes permanently. However, Mother Nature and her biological assistants are very clever. Even serious injuries can heal with little or no adverse effect and a decade or two later, it can be quite difficult to discern any diminution in function.

It may be impossible to convince an aggrieved claimant in the early phases of rehabilitation that such an outcome might eventuate.

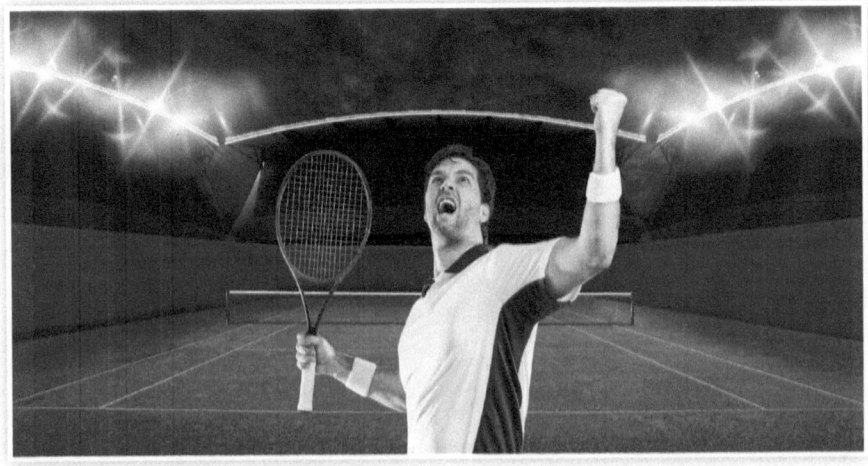

Understandably, the plaintiff and the plaintiff's legal advisor may express natural incredulity. However, it is the natural history of many injuries that near-normal function can be restored through competent treatment. In fairness to all who seek compensation at law for wrongful injury, it is only reasonable that the providers of compensation should be required to provide only to the extent of the long-term reality.

CASE VIGNETTE

Can You See The Funny Side?

Amidst all the sympathy for injured patients, an element of humour is sometimes present.

Two workers were on a construction site, dismantling a steel structure. It had two upright steel poles, about three metres apart, and extending about three metres above ground level. A third steel pole, affixed to the tops of the two upright poles, spanned the horizontal gap between them.

One worker was standing on a stepladder in the process of cutting the junction between one of the uprights and the horizontal beam. When the cut had been completed, the horizontal beam fell like a pendulum, as might be clearly expected. It struck the other worker heavily over his shoulder, causing a serious fracture-dislocation.

At the end of the consultation, he was asked why he was standing there. With a straight face, and without any hesitation, he said, "My boss told me to".

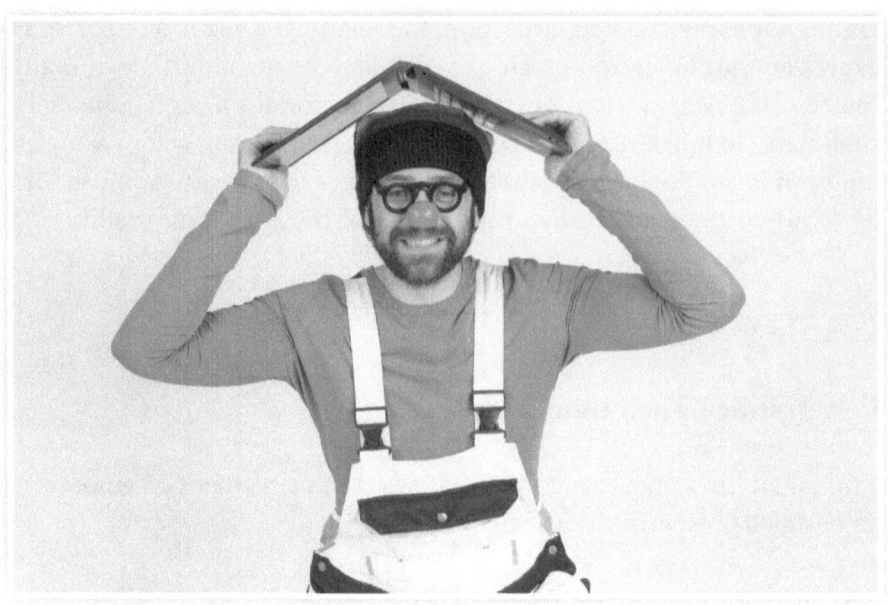

GENERAL ADVICE

Tell Them Not To Be Afraid.

Plaintiffs presenting for medicolegal examinations will have various expectations. Some think that the whole process may take several hours. Others will believe that the examiner will hurt them. A few won't know what to think. Not infrequently, patients express surprise that a thorough examination can be accomplished efficiently and without causing any great discomfort, perhaps because of poor prior experience.

It is possible to perform a thorough physical examination efficiently and almost painlessly. Careful attention to detail, being aware of patients' reactions and exercising proper professional skill can usually elicit all the necessary findings with a painless process.

LEAD ARTICLE

Traumatic Injuries Can Make You Mad

That does not connote a psychiatric or mental illness. Rather, they can be irritating frustrating, give rise to anger and anguish and generally make you cross. We all experience this from time to time, but some provocations are more provocative than others.

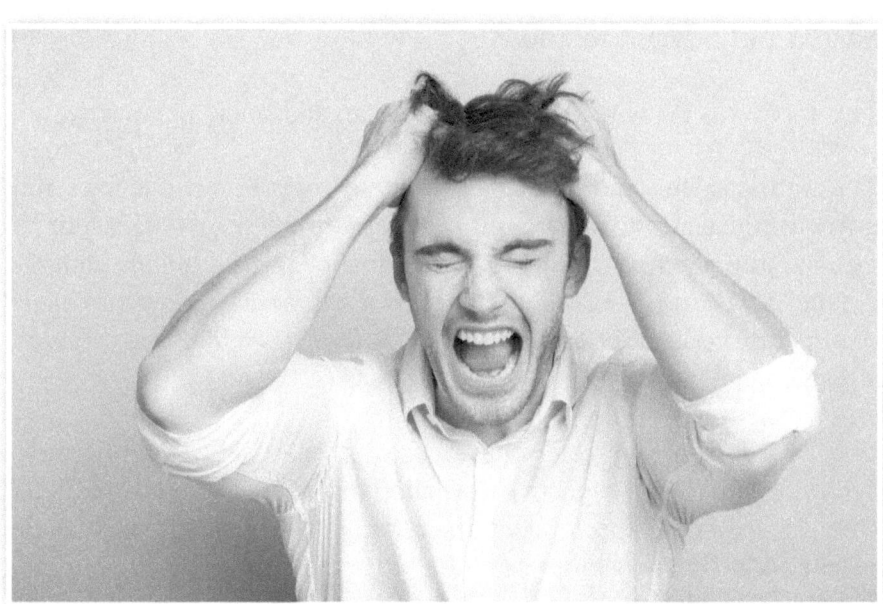

Can It Really Make You "Mad"?

There is another dimension. Consider a patient who has had an injury which follows a course contrary to the expected natural history. Whereas minor soft tissue injuries, strains and sprains typically heal quite promptly, this chap suffers a serious symptom complex five years later without tangible respite. It suggests that there is far more than just the simple physical condition involved.

Such patients may be emotionally altered, with some form of psychiatric illness. The relatively minor physical injury may have been the precipitant for a psychiatric response instead of a normal course of recovery. They present from time to time. It may assist to outline the medical reporter's views on the likely contribution of the physical injury to the circumstance, but also to recommend the need for psychiatric investigation and care. Typically, they do not return.

CASE VIGNETTE

Sexual Boundary Violations

This topic was canvassed earlier. This is an additional perspective.

The notifications committees of national registration agencies not infrequently deal with complaints of inappropriate sexual behaviour by medical practitioners towards patients. It appears that female patients are the most vulnerable, and that male practitioners are the more likely to offend. The severity and frequency of these violations vary, but all are anathema.

The Boards typically refer these cases to the Civil Administrative Tribunals in their respective jurisdictions. Respondents are dealt with according to the level of their breach, and sanctions include reprimands, suspensions or even cancellation of registrations, temporarily or indefinitely. In certain circumstances, criminal actions are also initiated by authorities.

Not only do the types of this violation cover a relatively broad spectrum, but there is also an added element in their potential for recidivism. Some practitioners have been dealt with on several occasions for the same violations and have been suspended, or otherwise allowed to practice, subject to the imposition of conditions, such as never to examine a female patient in the absence of a chaperone. It is surprising that there are still some practitioners who, despite repeated warnings, fail to adhere to the conditions set in place to protect society. Whatever the reason, every profession has them.

It appears that injured claimants are particularly vulnerable, and perhaps because an examination is usually conducted in isolation. The examiner may sense a power imbalance and take advantage of that situation. Perhaps, in suitable cases, claimants should be warned by their advocates to be on guard, since few patients would review public gazettes about medical practitioners for evidence of prior indiscretions.

GENERAL ADVICE

Qualities To Look For In An Expert

Some qualities may be considered desirable in medicolegal reporters. They include:

- Sufficient intellect, which is usually possessed by most medical practitioners. It may be associated with adequate education, especially in the subspecialty chosen.
- An analytical ability that allows the expert to sift through the evidence and make an accurate determination on issues of causation and loss.
- Adequate experience, both of and in, the subspecialty chosen.
- Erudition in reporting.
- An ability to maintain focus and communicate in a concise manner which includes expressing unequivocal decisions whenever possible, and with accompanying explanations.
- Remaining emotionless. Sometimes, reporters express frustration after dealing with a seemingly difficult plaintiff.

- Eliminating bias which is not always recognised by the reporter.
- Objectivity is paramount.
- Transparency is also essential. Conclusions and reasoning should always be explained.
- Completeness, always, with all questions answered, and factors that might be adverse to the opinion given revealed, with suitable discussion.

As the lawyers say, *"Res ipsa loquitur."* The principle is that the mere occurrence of some types of accident is insufficient to imply negligence.

A retired Justice of the Supreme Court of Queensland with considerable experience in medicolegal litigation and, as a former President of the Medical Tribunal, in medical discipline, has endorsed these proposals in their entirety. Special emphasis is placed on the need for completeness. If a report fully and fairly informs of all relevant features both for and against the opinion finally expressed, with an explanation for the preference, the trial judge can exercise his jurisdiction, and responsibility, properly. As a bonus, the reporter builds up treasures in Heaven as well as a sound reputation on Earth, even if the opinion is not accepted.

46

LEAD ARTICLE

Personality Does Matter

In two months, two plaintiffs alleged medical negligence against a "first surgeon". They had undergone total hip replacements by different surgeons. Let us call them surgeons A1 and A2. Both patients complained of ongoing discomfort. Amongst other things, it was alleged that leg length discrepancies had resulted, so great that they that both sought second opinions and underwent revision operations by, respectively, surgeons B1 and B2.

In fact, neither patient had a true leg length discrepancy. It was only an apparent one, and related to pelvic obliquity because of reversible abductor tightness, osteoarthritis in their contralateral hips and contralateral knees, and altered gait patterns. Although the osteoarthritic degeneration in their contralateral limbs could not be successfully treated easily, their gait patterns could have been quite easily resolved. The abductor muscles were destined to stretch, and the perceptions of limb lengthening would resolve spontaneously.

It was even more unfortunate that both operations performed by surgeons B1 and B2 were faulty. Considerable harm to both patients was caused during the revision procedures and, in the end, both were far worse than they might have been had they not been subjected to the revisions.

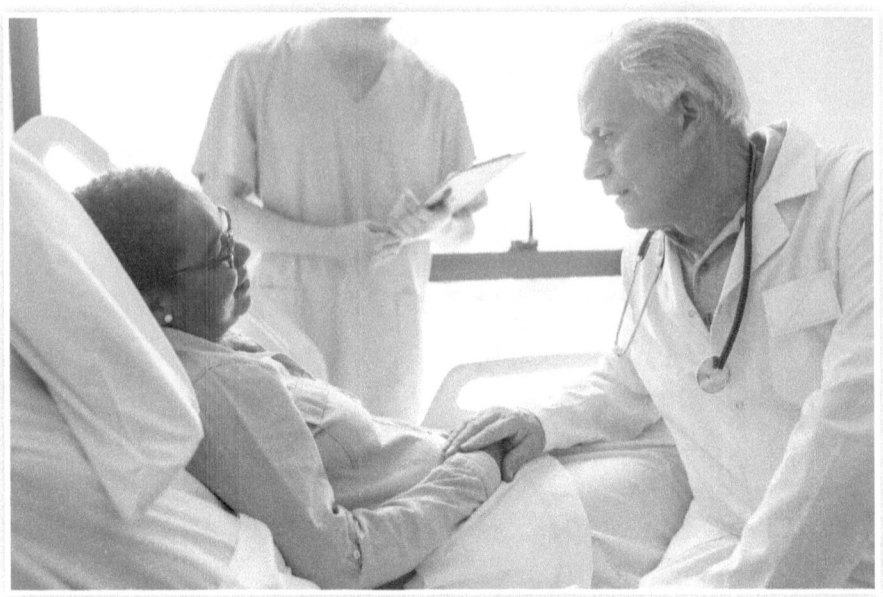

The respective patients had come to have total trust in Surgeon B1 and surgeon B2 and, through misdirection and misunderstanding, they sued surgeons A1 and A2. Suffice to say, after very large expenditure, many reports, and some clear-headed analysis, both suits failed.

CASE VIGNETTE

It's All A Matter Of Scale

A young man sustained a genuine injury in the region of his cervical spine while playing touch football at an Army base. It resulted in a discal protrusion, and he had an operative discectomy. As it sometimes happens, eight or nine months later, some of the remaining disc material that was not removed per-operatively protruded. The further extrusion was confirmed with a second MRI scan, and a second operation was performed. Unluckily, after a trivial incident at a restaurant, a third operation was required.

Next, he was involved in a rear end collision which might be described as relatively minor because he did not lose consciousness, the rear of his seat was not broken, the damage to the vehicle was less than AUD$1,000 and he was able to drive it from the scene of the accident for a further seven hours to a remote location. He claimed his baseline cervical spinal symptoms were increased by the collision and six or seven months later, he was subjected to a fourth operation in the form of a cervical fusion.

He brought an action against each of the Defence Force and the driver of the vehicle that had been involved in the collision. This required a medical division of the respective degrees of residual injury flowing from the alleged occasions of harm to which he had been subjected. It is always difficult to apportion blame accurately. To the defendants, it appeared that regardless of the rear end collision he was destined to require that fourth operation, and that it was of little or no significance to that result.

At The Trial

There was considerable disagreement amongst the expert witnesses. A neurosurgeon was adamant that this seemingly minor insult caused most of the patient's ongoing problems. The expert opined that the soldier had been coping satisfactorily before it occurred, and there was a definite change in his condition after it occurred. It was considered the principal precipitant in his requiring a fourth operation.

An orthopaedic witness took a contrary view. She explained that this was already a very vulnerable cervical spine from which the plaintiff was destined to suffer from ongoing pain indefinitely. The prior surgery had rendered at least one, and possibly two, mobile segments unstable. It was only a matter of time, and not long, before the fusion performed in the fourth operation would have been needed, even in the absence of this collision.

The court preferred the neurosurgical opinion, and the award, consisting of many components, was AUD$2.4 m.

GENERAL ADVICE

Fair Enough

Subject to ethical considerations, it is a lawyer's fundamental duty to take a client's side in controversial matters. It is in the interests of justice that each side should have the opportunity to present its case to the Court in the most efficient manner so that the Court will be apprised of the full facts and the best arguments as to the competing claims. For this, it is essential that each has the benefit of an expert lawyer who can advance its case in the best way. This can be achieved only if the lawyers engaged by the respective sides act in a way directed to that side's interests. Of course, in doing so, a competent lawyer will fully study the case of the other side, and its merits, and if those merits outweigh the merits of the client's case, the lawyer should inform the client of it and advise accordingly. It happens more than infrequently that a competent lawyer will act to the benefit of the Court and the other side, as well as to the client, by explaining to the client the desirability of discontinuing. Some firms specialise in acting either for the claimant or for the defendant. They wear such a role as a sign of competency in that class of work and bring to it expertise and efficiency.

One simple service of a plaintiff's lawyer may be to procure a report from a plaintiff-sympathetic expert, and that service is extended by not sending the client to a known unsympathetic expert. A defendant's lawyer might do the converse. It was said of one expert that he bore other people's pain with commendable fortitude. But such sympathy, or otherwise, is usually well-known to the Courts, which are usually very perspicacious in such matters, and a competent lawyer will usually prefer neutral competence that will be accepted by the Court.

The problem for such medical experts is that there are outlying colleagues who are exceedingly pro-plaintiff or pro-defendant. A report from one of these simply muddies the water. It confuses the accuracy of the middle ground, prolongs the matter, and adds to the cost of litigation. That may add to the fees of the legal firm, though not to the interests of a "no-win, no-fee" group.

Human nature weaves a rich tapestry of performance. Moral compasses sometimes drift. This issue is a complex matter. Raising it for public discussion and thus revealing it for what it is, is successful only if the voice is heard.

47

LEAD ARTICLE

Beware The Recidivist Claimant

Most persons will never bring a civil claim for personal injury. A small proportion will have one claim, and possibly two, though that would be unusual. Unsurprisingly, there is a tiny subset that lodges quite frequent claims. They appear to be extremely unlucky! Some will have been involved in six or seven collisions. Many will have frequently twisted an ankle, or both. Most of them seem to be skilled at relating the types of symptoms that purportedly add credence to their claim.

Dr Google has some part in it. Patients "surf" the internet to obtain the details of related symptomatology, have a good grasp on the natural history of the injury that would support it, and are even aware of the types of responses to investigations that are more believable than others.

Bias is an undesirable characteristic in an independent medical expert, but experience of such claims will often inform the expert towards serious caution. Plaintiffs with myriad antecedent civil claims for personal injury must arouse such reasonable caution.

CASE VIGNETTE

The Insults Some Plaintiffs Suffer

A young man had been working as a helicopter musterer on a remote cattle station for about eleven years. He was only thirty years of age when the helicopter he was flying crashed while executing dangerous manoeuvres through heavily wooded forest in search of the final beast or two for the complete muster. Fortunately, there was no fire though if there had been, its smoke may have attracted helpers to his aid more rapidly.

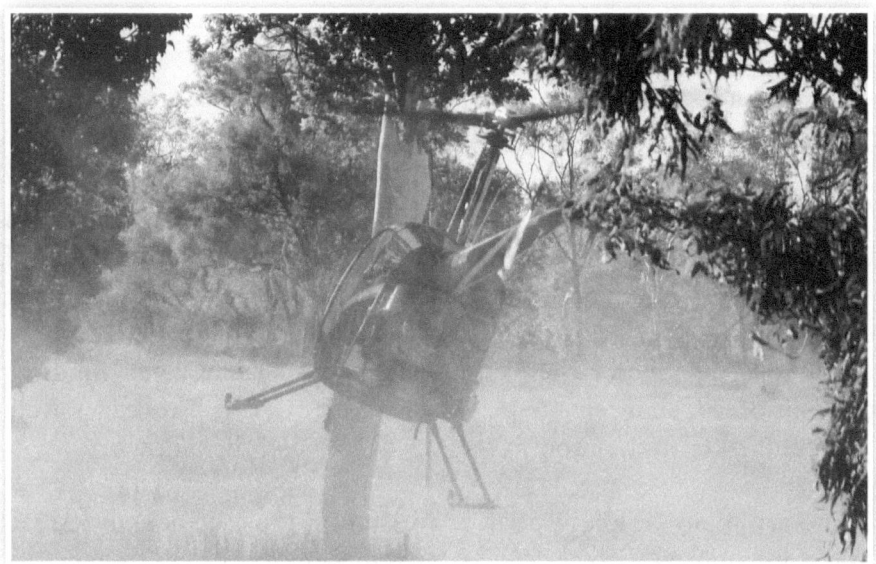

He sustained a severe thoracic spinal injury that rendered him completely paraplegic. He was able to use his upper limbs to drag himself from the wreckage and shelter beneath a tree. The accident occurred on dusk and the mid-winter night brought heavy dew and freezing cold. He realised the severity of his injury and genuinely believed that he was going to die. He nearly did. In that remote location, two full days elapsed before the alarm was raised and a rescue team found him. By then, his lower half was covered in excrement, he had been severely bitten by ants, and he was delirious with hunger and thirst. Even after many months of rehabilitation, his physical and emotional turmoil abounded. Extraordinary challenges hampered his progress and the lives of those close to him were altered permanently.

At his medicolegal examination, four years later, his face was suntanned, his upper limbs were strong and equally tanned, he was relaxed, focused, balanced and in control. He was accompanied by his wife of seven years. Though he was confined to a wheelchair, it seemed that most other facets of his life were restored.

His response to adversity, his desire to make the best of what was available to him, and the partnership he had forged with his wife were all remarkable. It offered a new perspective on personal problems.

GENERAL ADVICE

The Plight Of The Insured Worker

The principal problem of claimants for worker's compensation is the perceived inadequacy of the offer. A disturbingly familiar list of accompanying complaints includes difficulties in contacting their counsellor by telephone because messages are left unattended for days, a lack of sympathy for their circumstance, especially when finances are considered, being sent to medicolegal reporters who are excessively gruff and rude, and a process that tends to grind them down.

There are many different perspectives and it must be acknowledged that some injured workers can be extremely demanding. To generate a level of compassion for them all, it is fair to recognise that, had it not been for the accident, which is often not their fault, they would not have been in their unhappy situation. They feel anger, frustration, and a sense of helplessness.

Part of the problem lies with the bureaucracy of public servants, a few of whom lack dedication, drive and determination to secure a fair outcome for the client. There is sometimes a culture of unjustified disbelief in the genuineness of claims, and little recognition of the urgency required for a response. Statutory guidelines cap payments, and though injured workers are better without nothing, the *status quo* remains inadequate.

It is difficult to suggest a panacea, but some modest compassion from a medical assessor could help towards smoothing the turbulent waters of discontent.

48

LEAD ARTICLE

What's The Difference Between The Heart And The Brain?

From the medical perspective, there are very significant differences between these two important organs. From the legal perspective, the terms are used a little more loosely. The heart is often regarded in sympathetic terms as softer, and a source of compassion, while the brain is regarded as the intellectual motor, harder and more calculating. From a medicolegal perspective, it is necessary to engage the brain to report without the influence of emotion. The goal is transparency, objectivity and correctness.

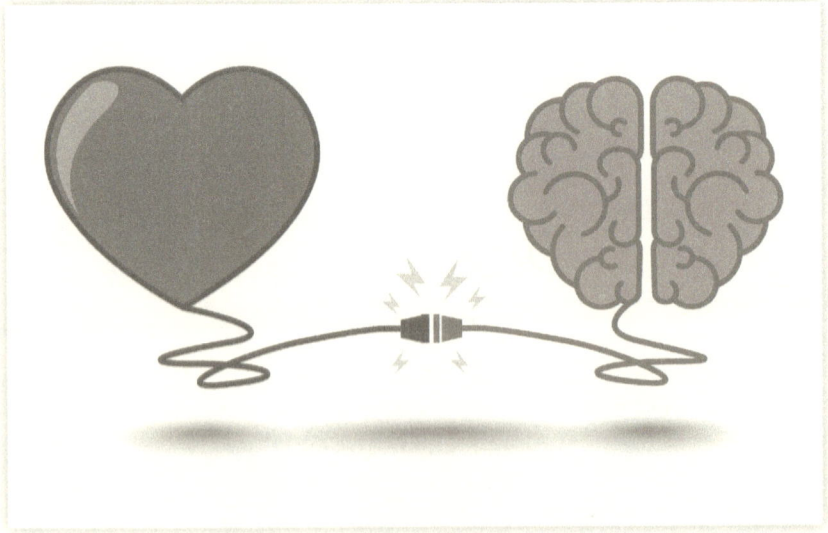

There are times when a reporter's heart might have a report framed differently, particularly on the issue of causation of the patient's permanent residue of symptoms or disability. Some patients will have been very seriously injured, and the course of their lives irreversibly altered for the worse. Unfortunately, if the cause is not as they believe, it may have a non-compensable status at law. It is then tempting to adopt a more lenient view, but that might be both wrong and potentially immoral. Then, it can only be hoped that the law will be found to be different.

The written word can be very persuasive. Words can also convey sensitivity with facts. Discerning readers will detect a deeper message in carefully crafted opinions. We can only hope.

CASE VIGNETTE

I Sometimes Change My Mind

Prior to seeing a patient regarding injuries that are the basis of a personal injury claim, a reporter at least scans the briefed documentation. It generally includes hospital and medical notes, records from the patient's general practitioner, and, importantly, specialty notes and reports, There will be some likelihood that the reporter will form a provisional impression about the matter before seeing the patient. It is not unreasonable, since the judgment is provisional only.

On such occasions, after taking a full history, performing a thorough physical examination and reviewing the ancillary investigations, the reporter's mind is frequently changed, sometimes to the opposite view. There may be many reasons, including the inability of some of the previously reporting experts to have had access to all the relevant data, misinterpretation of data, a failure to glean a proper history, and the basing of opinions on misapprehensions, from whatever source.

This experience may be very refreshing, and it is a source of satisfaction to have had an open mind. Being able to acknowledge the need to "change one's mind" is a strength.

GENERAL ADVICE

Reasonable Fees

Medical negligence cases typically involve reams and reams, or gigabytes and gigabytes. of material to decipher, digest and analyse carefully. Properly performed, it may take many hours.

Some solicitors, typically those acting for plaintiffs, wish to receive verbal advice before a written report is formally sought. They may not risk potentially receiving a damaging report which they may be required to disclose to the defendant's side, made more powerful because it would have come from the plaintiff's side. Nonetheless, even in those circumstances the expert is still required to spend all those hours reviewing the evidence, distilling the facts carefully, and formulating a reliable opinion, even if it is to be given verbally. The solicitor, therefore, should expect that there will be a bill for this service.

An interstate solicitor failed to pay an account for such services for nine months. His initial excuse was that their telephone conversation had lasted for only 11 minutes, which conveniently ignored the hours that had been spent in preparation. His final flourish was that the expert must have known that the opinion was not going to support his client and, therefore, there was no justification for charging for the service. The first excuse is redolent of that in a famous action taken by the artist, Whistler, against an aristocrat whose portrait Whistler had painted. To the defendant's Queen's Counsel who had cross-examined, "Mr. Whisler, you are claiming five hundred guineas for three day's work?", he responded, "Yes, and thirty years of study and experience!"

Medicolegal experts are engaged to assess the entire truth, if it is available, and to give an honest, objective, transparent and most practical of all, defendable opinion. Whether it is helpful to the client or not, the instructing solicitor should still pay the fee.

LEAD ARTICLE

Mandatory Reporting

At a dinner of members of both the legal and medical professions, three speakers, all from different backgrounds, dealt with the topic of mandatory reporting. The lawyer, who was engaged by the medical defence organization, was excellently concise, erudite, focused, objective and educational. Her performance was faultless.

There Were Two Central Issues

The **first** related to the mandate. If a medical practitioner has a reasonable belief that a fellow practitioner is under-performing, engaging in unprofessional conduct, or is guilty of professional misconduct, it must be reported. Simply stated though this may be, it has its ambiguities. One question could be how to define "reasonable"? A lawyer would say that it is the understanding of an ordinary person in the position of, and with the knowledge of, the person concerned, and certainly not that of the person concerned. The understanding of that hypothetical person might still be debatable is some circumstances, but it seems that no-one has ever been castigated for a frivolous or vexatious notification under this mandatory reporting system. Of course, that does not exclude the existence of an excessive unwillingness to report. Some may fear that to report might be viewed as anti-competitive behaviour.

Nevertheless, if a practitioner reasonably believes that another is behaving in the proscribed way, there is a legal obligation to report it, rather than to adjudicate on it. After all, a practitioner's principal focus should be on the welfare of patients. The accrediting authority will take the matter in hand, and deal with the report fairly, justly and transparently. If a report can be justified as something that is honestly believed, rather than, say, something based upon jealousy, it might be expected to be reasonably safe. If there is any doubt, recourse to legal advice would be wise.

Two operating theatre nurses approached a specialist, complaining about their concern at the performance of one of his colleagues. Both expressed their thoughts in writing, and the practitioner simply passed it on to the state registration agency, without repercussions.

The **second** issue related to detecting and establishing the under-performance, unprofessional conduct or professional misconduct. Theoretically, this may be more difficult, but in practice, it should not be so. Some may find the process taxing, but that might be merely a matter of competence in the investigator since it is an alien field. Importantly, is must not dissuade the mandated reporting.

CASE VIGNETTE

How Much Is An Injury Worth?

A youngish woman of thirty-three was bumped by a horse and fell, not awkwardly, onto soft lawn. It really did not involve much trauma. No doubt, it was a little frightening, but she had an anxious disposition, was embarrassed, and began to cry inconsolably. She later sued the horse owner and, over the following three years, sought advice and treatment from medical practitioners from almost every specialty.

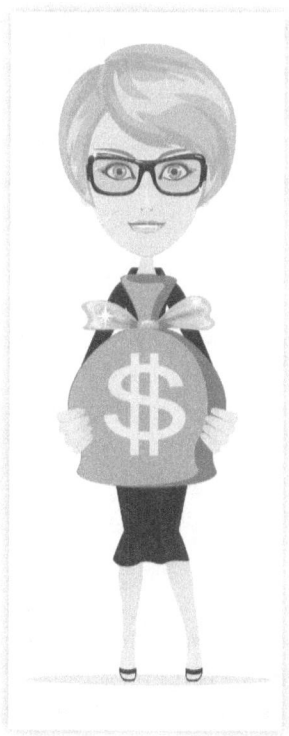

She had a prior history of back problems. Her plane radiographs showed wear and tear slightly more than her age would suggest. A sympathetic medical expert gave her a supportive opinion on causation and impairment, and she was awarded $630,000 in her civil action.

The insurer appealed. It was alleged insufficient attention was paid to her past history, inadequate allowance for made for the trivial nature of the insult, and her claims of remunerative incapacity were not substantiated. The appeal was successful. The award was reduced significantly and the costs for the appeal were awarded to the applicant.

GENERAL ADVICE

Who Is Responsible?

A thirty year old diesel fitter jumped from the rear of a Caterpillar bulldozer and landed awkwardly some 85 cm below on uneven ground.

He sustained a twisting injury to his left ankle. It was probably an inversion injury whereby the foot is turned inwards and the structures on the outside, the lateral side, of the ankle joint can be strained, sprained or even torn. In this case, it was a relatively minor sprain injury. A MRI scan examination confirmed that all the structures were still intact, although there was some local bruising around the anterior talofibular ligament.

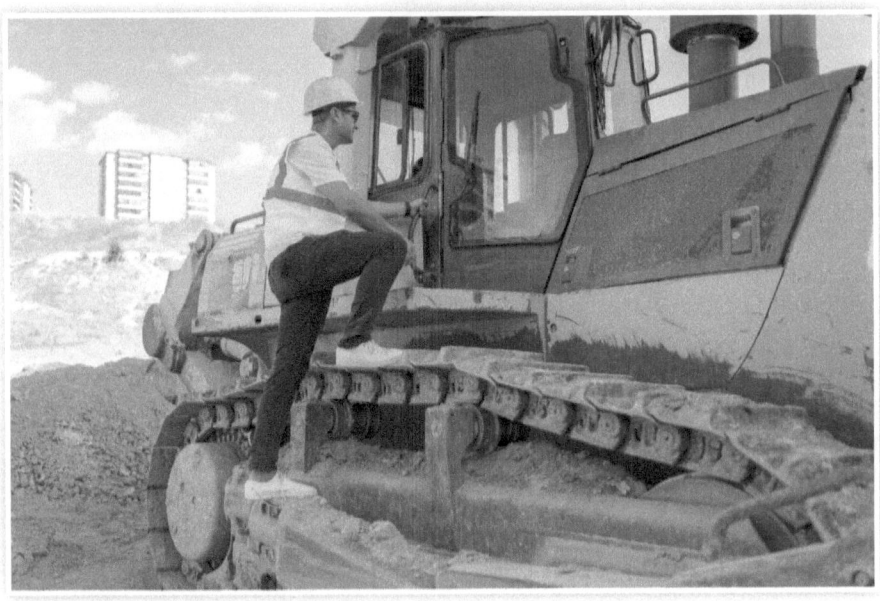

The natural history for this type of injury is for gradual healing. Most patients return to symptomatic normality within the following six to twelve months, and many do so much more quickly. Unfortunately, he was referred to an orthopaedic surgeon who operated early, rather than allowing nature to take its course. It led to no improvement, but rather, to a worsening of the patient's condition. There was a primary wound infection which in turn invaded his ankle joint proper. This gave rise to dissolution or destruction of the cartilage within the joint, and quite severe secondary post-infection arthritis developed. The sural nerve, which supplies sensation to the lateral side of the foot and the lateral two or three toes, was also damaged irretrievably. This combination of a stiff, painful, swollen ankle joint and a numb lateral border of the foot, with associated burning or dysaesthesia, made the patient very much more disabled than he might have been.

When he made his claim for damages, the reviewing medicolegal reporters all agreed on several points. The original injury was quite minor and did not require operative intervention. Had he not been subjected to an operation it was highly probable that he would have made a complete recovery. His ongoing circumstance was simply an extension of the inappropriateness of the orthopaedic operative intervention.

Practitioners all have varying responsibilities. Expert medical reporters have a duty to identify the medical facts, to tell the truth and leave no gaps. The use that is made of a report is a matter for the patient's lawyers. This minor workplace injury morphed into a medical negligence claim.

There is a lesson. Whether choosing your surgeon for clinical attention or a medicolegal reporter, do so wisely.

50

Some readers skip to the ending of a book and read it first. Others proceed through a publication sequentially and read the final chapter at the conclusion.

Well, I am ready for you both!

To the former, expect an eclectic mix of experience, both true and borrowed. Those that are true have been deidentified beyond recognition. If you think you see yourself, you are wrong. The same can be said for that which has been borrowed. Every segment has a message and possibly a lesson. If it becomes educational, understand that it has been written with humility. Perceived wisdom has grown from errors. The package is complete, yet random. You can start and finish anywhere, anytime. Juxtaposition of thoughts adds to the journey. You are not being led, cajoled or coerced. I encourage you to pause and reflect. Mull issues over. Test opinions. Become a traveler on the journey.

To those of you who have lasted the distance, run the race and stuck with me, I am grateful. Regardless of your profession, there will be many cases, examples, successes and failures that will revive vivid memories. Together we have explored a fascinating niche of medicine and law. I hope that the tips, tricks and trials resonate usefully. You too might recognise someone you think you know. Gosh, you might even sense yourself. Be reassured. Likenesses are serendipitous. Causing offence is excluded from this work.

We share a fascinating professional interest. Some of you, like me, will have been an injured plaintiff. Receiving a just and fair outcome would be warmly welcomed. Every claimant will find something of solace between these pages.

Legal practitioners occupy a special position in the sequence. Assessing the merits of a claim, assuming the responsibility of carriage, making correct decisions at the right time, and serving your client are equally challenging, and rewarding.

Medical practitioners are invitees into the domain, unless the subject of a claim. Characteristics of calm, collectedness, objectivity and lucidity form part of the necessary tapestry. It can be a most satisfying part of a professional career.

The judiciary remains indispensable for many reasons. Most dear to me is the single focus of decision making. With that privilege comes great responsibility. We can all assist.

And finally, good night.

ACKNOWLEDGEMENTS

I applaud the tradition of acknowledging assistance when it has been offered and provided. No work of this nature can materalise from the ether. Contacts and liaisons with numerus colleagues and mentors in medicine and law have molded me, provided professional sustenance, and engendered balance in all I do. To all of you, I offer my sincere gratitude.

Naming individuals is fraught with danger. The risk of inadvertently missing someone, overlooking another or completely forgetting a third fills me with horror. With that in mind, I have two exceptions.

The first is the Honourable Desmond Derrington, retired Supreme Court Justice and the author of the Foreword. He has been a constant source of education and support for decades. He has also proofread this book and provided expert advice. He has been a father, a brother and a friend.

The second is Christine Bowker. She has been our practice manager for nearly forty years and has created, crafted, nurtured and sustained every nuance in this publication. Her honesty, loyalty, competence and unswerving support have made it possible. I am eternally grateful.

Wherever you are, I thank you.

www.ingramcontent.com/pod-product-compliance
Lightning Source LLC
Chambersburg PA
CBHW020632220526
45464CB00001B/112